THE RAW FOOD REVOLUTION DIET

feast · lose weight · gain energy · feel younger

by Cherie Soria, Brenda Davis, RD, and Vesanto Melina, MS, RD

BOOK PUBLISHING COMPANY

Summertown, Tennessee

Library of Congress Cataloging-in-Publication Data

Soria, Cherie, 1947-
   The raw food revolution diet : feast, lose weight, gain energy,
feel younger! / by Cherie Soria, Brenda Davis, and Vesanto Melina.
      p. cm.
   Includes bibliographical references and index.
   ISBN 978-1-57067-185-2 (alk. paper)
   1. Raw food diet. 2. Nutrition. I. Davis, Brenda, 1959- II.
Melina, Vesanto, 1942- III. Title.

   RM237.5.S67 2008
   613.2'6—dc22

                                                     2008012247

Pictured on the front cover, from left:

canapés, made with Almond Nut Cheese, p. 136, and Sun-Dried Tomato Tapenade, p. 139

Apples and Walnuts on Baby Greens with Poppy Seed Dressing, p. 179

Zoom Burgers, p. 208, and Crispy Sweet Onion Rings, p. 134, with Cashew Mayonnaise, p. 166, Hot Mustard, p. 167, and Real Tomato Ketchup, p. 168

Garden Pizza, p. 202, using Sprouted Seed Pizza Crusts, p. 132, Pizza Sauce, p. 161, and Almond Cheese, p. 136

parfaits, using Cashew Yogurt, p. 108

© 2008 Cherie Soria, Brenda Davis, Vesanto Melina

Cover and interior design: *Aerocraft Charter Art Service*
Cover and interior photos: *Dan Ladermann*
Illustrations: *Matt Gouig*

Printed in Canada

Book Publishing Company
P.O. Box 99
Summertown, TN 38483
888-260-8458
www.bookpubco.com

ISBN 13: 978-1-57067-185-2

17 16 15 14 13 12 11 10 09   3 4 5 6 7 8 9 10

Book Publishing Co. is a member of Green Press Initiative. We chose to print this title on paper with postconsumer recycled content, processed without chlorine, which saved the following natural resources:

111 trees

4,713 pounds of solid waste

40,418 gallons of water

8,935 pounds of greenhouse gases

78 million BTUs of total energy

For more information, visit www.greenpressinitiative.org.

(Paper calculations from Environmental Defense Paper Calculator, www.edf.org/papercalculator)

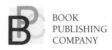

BOOK PUBLISHING COMPANY

green press INITIATIVE

contents

acknowledgments

Sincere gratitude to all those at the Book Publishing Company who made this book possible:

- Our dear publisher, Bob Holzapfel; our wonderful editors, Cynthia Holzapfel and Jo Stepaniak; and the talented staff, Warren Jefferson and Anna Pope.

Love and gratefulness to our dear families and loved ones:

- Cherie's husband, business partner, and right arm, Dan Ladermann, and her dear parents, Fred and Georgette Soria, who have been a great inspiration and support throughout her life.
- Brenda's beloved husband, Paul, and her amazing children, Leena and Cory.
- Vesanto's dear partner, Cam Doré, son Chris, and daughter Kavyo, each of whom means so very much to her.

Deepest appreciation to our cherished advisors, mentors, and colleagues:

- Cherie's mentors Viktoras Kulvinskas and Dr. Ann Wigmore, and her dearest friend, Terri Zacanti, who has shared her raw food journey.
- Eternal blessings to all those who contributed recipes and tested recipes, including Martine Lussier, Jennifer Cornbleet, Elaina Love, and Brooke Peterson.
- Much gratitude to Cherie's friends Laurie Masters, Christina Chadney, and Jeannie Moffitt for their help preparing this manuscript, as well as the supportive staff at Living Light International, especially Kristin Suratt, Julie Engfer, and Patricia Hoskins.
- Vesanto's wonderful and supportive friends and neighbors at WindSong Cohousing Community who have enthusiastically tested recipes and "gone green."
- Brenda's cherished friend, Margie Colclough, who assisted with testing and provided many hours of support and encouragement.

Sincerest thanks to our treasured friends:

- Margie Roswell for her generous and kind financial support for the nutritional analysis of Green Giant Juice and certain raw ingredients.
- Vesanto's friend Sooze Waldock, for whom raw foods have proven to be such a healing force.
- Friend and consultant David Ross, who recommended we write this book.
- Excalibur Inc.
- Sam Young Photography.

We want to thank the following people for their recipe contributions:

- Living Light chef instructors Matt Samuelson for Zucchini Hummus (page 145) and for the inspiration for Hot Lava Sauce (page 171), Elaina Love for Baby Bok Choy with Shiitake Mushrooms (page 197), and Patricia Hoskins for Minestrone Italiano (page 190).
- Living Light associate chefs Amy Greenebaum for Creamy Hemp Dressing (page 149) and Amy Wells for her collaboration on Spicy Papaya Soup (page 192).
- Alicia Ojeda for Sprouted Seed Pizza Crusts (page 132).
- Liquid Gold Dressing (page 151) is adapted from the nutrition books *The New Becoming Vegetarian* and *Becoming Vegan*, both by Brenda Davis and Vesanto Melina (Book Publishing Company 2003, 2000) and *Raising Vegetarian Children*, by Jo Stepaniak and Vesanto Melina (McGraw-Hill 2003).
- Felix Schoner for assistance with food styling, pictured on page 135 and the cover.

foreword

The *Raw Food Revolution Diet* is an exciting and intelligent contribution to the most important dietary trend of the twenty-first century. The authors' astute and inspiring presentation is grounded in their commonsense approach. Cherie Soria has been a primary impetus behind the global dissemination of knowledge about the preparation and consumption of high-frequency foods. Vesanto Melina, MS, RD, and Brenda Davis, RD, contribute the nutrition science that supports this healing and health-promoting way of life. Raw food is not only beautiful and delectable, it also contains the vital nutrients that afford each cell the fuel it requires to function optimally.

These three great minds weave together a refreshing, lucid, and highly accessible publication. The Raw Food Revolution Diet is not a concept, it is a reality. There are millions of people around the world who have successfully and joyfully adopted this way of eating and are reaping the multitude of benefits, from slowing the aging process to preventing and healing disease.

Over the last 30 years, I have had the privilege of directing the Hippocrates Health Institute. For more than half a century, Hippocrates has guided hundreds of thousands of people back to health by teaching them how to enjoy raw and living cuisine. Our decades of clinical research have shattered the common fallacies about diet and health. Today there is no doubt that all serious nutritional scientists encourage the use of raw and living food to help their clients in their quest to achieve superior health.

Recently, Europe hosted the largest conference ever held on the topic of antiaging. After days of intriguing presentations about alternative therapies, exciting treatments, and innovative approaches, the president of the event concluded, "At the heart of preventing premature aging is the use of organic, raw, vegan living food." *The Raw Food Revolution Diet* is a road map for anyone who wants improved health and greater longevity. I am honored to introduce this work and encourage you to pass it on to those you love.

Brian R. Clement, PhD

THE RAW FOOD DIET—IT'S A REVOLUTION

There's a revolution going on all over the world! Throughout Europe, Asia, and the Americas; in places like Australia and New Zealand; even in countries like Greenland, Iceland, Saudi Arabia, and South Africa, this revolution is creating a groundswell of interest in health and well-being on all levels of body, mind, and spirit.

Revolution occurs when people have had enough of the status quo and the effect it has on their personal freedom or way of life. Today, many of us are sick and tired of being sick and tired! We are quietly rebelling against traditional medicine and are actively seeking out alternatives. We no longer want to be victims of poor health and obesity and are convinced it's time to take our health into our own hands.

It's unfortunate that the profound relationship between food and health is not reflected in most medical school curriculums. Nutrition is not always a mandatory course, and its relevance to health is largely underrated. Many physicians don't practice healthful lifestyle habits themselves and are ill equipped to promote such changes to their patients. All too often, the potential for diet and lifestyle intervention as a serious treatment option is ignored. Unfortunately, our medical system is better set up to support physicians in filling out prescriptions for expensive medications with potentially damaging side effects. Many of us have lost faith in the promise that prescription drugs are our best bet for treating disease and are concerned that physicians are in the back pocket of the pharmaceutical industry. We're becoming better educated about the dangers of conventional food production and its consequences on our health, the health of our children, and the health of our planet.

This revolution of consciousness is happening all over the globe, the result of which is that humanity is discovering the benefits of the Raw Food Revolution Diet. This revolution supports a natural way of living that can enable us to feel in control of our lives in a way that most of us have never experienced. The Raw Food Revolution Diet fosters not only the health and well-being of humanity, it preserves the well-being of the creatures of the earth and, indeed, the earth itself.

If you are overweight and seeking permanent weight loss, or just want to achieve better health and more energy, there is a simple, natural way to bring your body into balance without giving up the enjoyment of delicious, satisfying, nurturing meals. That's correct—you can lose weight, gain energy, and feel younger while feasting on foods that nourish your body and delight your senses! The Raw Food Revolution Diet, with its emphasis on sensible, plant-based nutrition, offers what no other weight-loss diet can: it helps you bring your weight into balance while you become healthier and happier simultaneously. This is a diet you can live with even after you've reached your weight-loss goals. In fact, you may find that you feel so much better on the Raw Food Revolution Diet (like others who have tried this approach to health and weight loss) that you are motivated to stay on it and maintain your new, slender, healthier, more energetic self for the rest of your life. Get off the weight loss/weight gain merry-go-round—forever!

The Raw Food Revolution Diet does not require that you count calories, eliminate carbohydrates, or throw your body out of balance by eating too much protein—nor does it require that you give up familiar comfort foods. On the contrary, it is a delicious, satisfying, plant-based diet that is loaded with the nutrients you need to fight disease and become more vital. The Raw Food Revolution Diet delivers a bounty of the nutrients the human body requires in order to be optimally healthy: protein, vitamins, minerals, phytochemicals, antioxidants, and carotenoids.

The best part is you can meet your daily nutritional requirements without feeling deprived. You can enjoy burgers with all the trimmings, burritos, chips and dips, and even (nondairy) ice cream. Are you still not sure you can be satisfied on a raw food diet? Then spend a week or so eating more raw fruits and vegetables than you typically do, plus a big green salad every day, along with many of your usual foods. Then, try the Raw Food Revolution Diet described in this book for 21 days; you'll be amazed at how good you look and feel!

At Living Light Culinary Arts Institute, we've been teaching people about nutritious, delicious, vegan and raw food meals since 1997, and in that time we have worked with thousands of people who have reached their weight-loss goals and sustained this weight loss, in excellent health, using the Raw Food Revolution Diet. Even people who appear to be healthy and are not overweight report increased energy, a greater sense of well-

Some of the Many Benefits of The Raw Food Revolution Diet

- improved health and general well-being
- weight loss and weight maintenance
- increased energy, stamina, and vitality
- less sleep required
- fewer or complete elimination of allergies, colds, and flus
- more positive attitude
- better digestion
- disease prevention and reversal
- less addictive behavior
- protection of animals and the environment

being, and a more youthful appearance. Nothing is more important than your mental, physical, and spiritual well-being—and all of these are dependent on maintaining a healthy body weight and eating foods that not only meet your daily nutrient requirements, but are emotionally satisfying, too. The Raw Food Revolution Diet provides all of this and more. It's a diet for life.

USING THIS BOOK TO REVOLUTIONIZE YOUR LIFE

The Raw Food Revolution Diet provides many ideas and suggestions to assist you in the preparation of simple, delicious foods to suit your lifestyle, time constraints, and taste preferences. This is a moderate approach, created to inspire and assist those interested in losing weight and becoming healthier and more conscious about their food choices. Even if you only increase the raw plant-based foods in your daily diet by 10%, you'll be doing that much better at meeting your weight-loss goals and will probably feel the difference. We provide scientific information that will explain the benefits of the Raw Food Revolution Diet and prove to you that this is the most sensible weight-loss diet there is.

You'll find guidance for setting up and managing your raw food kitchen. To help eliminate the guesswork, there's a list of foods and equipment you may want to have on hand to make food preparation easier and more fun. We'll show you how to stock your pantry and ripen and store fruits and vegetables for optimal nutrition. You'll learn how to sprout and how to plan menus that support your weight-loss goals. Shopping and food preparation guides are provided to make it easy for you to follow the weight-loss menus on pages 92–100. There are even tips about how to travel and still follow the Raw Food Revolution Diet.

Finally, you'll find over 150 fabulous, well-tested, raw food recipes. Some are the essence of simplicity and others are true gourmet fare. Although most of our recipes are 100% raw, a few use minor or optional ingredients that are not raw (such as vanilla extract); this makes it easy for you to create treats that are as good or better than the ones you have been accustomed to.

Now—start losing excess weight and enjoying excellent health, energy, and vitality for a lifetime!

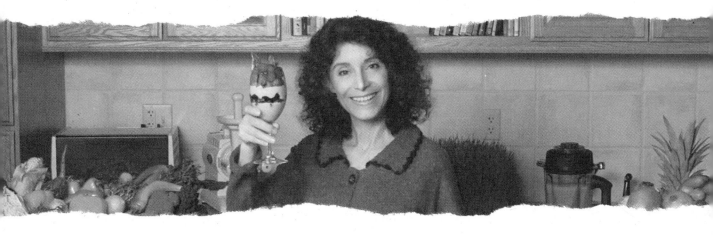

introduction

OUR SUCCESS STORIES

Cherie: *How I Became a Raw Food Revolutionary*

Chronic illness and a family history of heart disease and cancer motivated me, at an early age, to study everything I could find about health and the cause of disease. I saw family members who had been slender as young-sters who later became obese and developed diabetes, heart problems, and other diet-related, potentially life-threatening diseases. I wanted to escape the writing on the wall that promised either cancer, heart disease, or some other form of "death sentence" that was likely to rob me of a life of health and vitality. This led me to embrace a vegetarian diet in my early twenties and to teach others about its benefits.

I have always been a gifted chef—in fact, I won my first cooking con-test at the age of 12. By the time I discovered the raw food diet, I was 44 years old and had been teaching vegetarian culinary arts for nearly 20 years. During that time, I evolved from eating fried soybean burgers with dairy cheese and egg-based mayonnaise to eating low-fat, baked veggie burgers with soy cheese and vegan mayo. In those days my diet was con-sidered extreme, but the colds and flus that had plagued me in my youth virtually disappeared and I felt great. I became active and athletic, was an avid skier and tennis player, and even earned a black belt in karate. I looked and felt great and had maintained my girlish figure.

Even so, I continued to study about health and was always looking for more information that would help me enjoy perpetual youth of mind, body, and spirit. I learned that there are many factors that contribute to disease, and diet is an important key. Then, in 1990, I read a book called *Be Your Own Doctor*, by a remarkable woman named Ann Wigmore, who had healed herself and was healing others of life-threatening illnesses using only raw plant-based foods. Even though I had no health challenges, this fascinated me, so I decided to spend my vacation at her clinic in Puerto Rico to learn more.

When I first went to the Ann Wigmore Natural Health Institute, I was simply curious to meet Ann Wigmore and to see firsthand what she was doing and how it affected people. I also wanted to experience how a diet of 100% raw food would affect me, although at the time I thought of it more as a cleansing program than as a lifestyle. I certainly had no intention of changing my life or giving up the popular vegetarian and vegan cooking classes I had been teaching for two decades. I truthfully never considered continuing to eat a raw food diet when I returned home.

However, what I witnessed at the Institute changed my life forever. While I was there, a man with cancer received a clean bill of health from the same doctor who had only months before told him to go home and put his affairs in order! I saw a woman who arrived there unable to walk up the stairs but was able to run on the beach two short weeks later. Another woman, who was chronically depressed, left with a new lease on life, happy to be truly alive for the first time in 20 years.

Some people just went to the institute to lose weight, and they succeeded. Many of them had been there before and had to keep coming back, because they couldn't stay on the strict, tasteless diet we were served at the clinic. The food included all the wheatgrass juice one could drink and a blended concoction of fruits and sprouts for lunch and dinner. On occasion, we were given something like a salad that we could actually chew! Even without salt, garlic, or onion for flavor, it was considered a treat. The food was not intended to be tasty, and I knew it was not something that most people would enjoy on a daily basis. But after spending time with Ann Wigmore and seeing the "miraculous" weight-loss and healing effects of her program, I decided that I would devote myself to developing delicious, raw, dairy-free vegetarian cuisine that people could enjoy every day for the rest of their lives.

I particularly set my sights on creating comfort foods, so meals could be health promoting, delicious, and familiar. After teaching for nearly 20 years, I knew that people wanted food to feed their emotions as much as their bodies, so even though Ann Wigmore's simple raw foods could help sick, overweight people lose weight and become healthier, I feared they would become too bored to continue eating the way they were being fed at the institute. That meant they would most likely soon return to their old ways, gain their weight back, and develop health problems once again.

I returned home motivated to develop what is now known as gourmet raw vegan cuisine. At the time, I didn't know of anyone who was making raw food that was anything more than glorified salads, smoothies, simple nut pâtés, juices, and unpalatable blended green soups. Some people might find that these provide enough variety, but the vast majority of us want the familiar foods we grew up with. With my culinary talent, I knew I could create delicious foods that everybody would enjoy.

During that time, I ate only raw food and found I was not attracted to the cooked foods I had loved so much before. In fact, much to my surprise, I found myself requiring far less sleep and feeling tremendously more energetic throughout the day. My hair became thicker and people told me I looked younger and more radiant. I felt a greater connection to the world around me and a deeper sense of spirituality than I had ever experienced before. In fact, even though I had no health problems, was not overweight, and was physically fit due to my years as a vegetarian, this dietary change was by far the most profound transformation I had ever experienced. I found it truly creative and exciting to be designing a new culinary art that was delicious and satisfying, and I started teaching classes to my culinary students, who were interested in what I was now up to.

Over the next two years my energy and mental clarity continued to improve, and friends who hadn't seen me in years commented that I seemed to keep getting younger. I even went through menopause without the usual mood swings and hot flashes that many other women complained about. I continued to teach classes in raw culinary arts and saw that most of my students were also experiencing these profound improvements in their health and well-being.

I wanted to encourage others to add more raw food to their diets, so I wrote a book that included over 125 gourmet raw recipes and an equal number of cooked, nondairy vegetarian recipes. The book reflected my newfound spiritual connection, so I called it *Angel Foods: Healthy Recipes for Heavenly Bodies.* The recipes it included not only made people feel good, they were delicious and emotionally satisfying. I never suggested that people give up their favorite cooked foods—I simply showed them how to make delicious meals that didn't require cooking.

I started teaching this revolutionary gourmet raw vegan cuisine at international vegetarian organizations, and in 1997, I started the first raw vegan culinary school, Living Light Culinary Arts Institute. To my surprise, people came from all over the world to learn how to prepare this new cuisine. Many of my students have gone on to write raw recipe books and open restaurants. But what has meant the most to me are the letters I have received from those whose lives have been transformed as a result of eating raw food.

Since I started Living Light, thousands of people have attended my chef training classes. The majority of those who were overweight lost that weight at the rate of about 10 pounds over a two- to three-week period. Many of them also experienced a radical transformation in their personal and professional lives, much of it the result of how the weight loss and energy gain helped them to feel more empowered and more connected to themselves and the world around them.

This is why I realized that a book dedicated to showing people how to lose weight or just gain energy and feel younger without giving up great-tasting food would be a valuable tool. I felt compelled to prove that a raw vegan diet is safe for the majority of the adult population, so I enlisted two women whom I regard highly in the field of health and nutrition, Vesanto Melina and Brenda Davis, both registered dietitians and authors. When I first approached Vesanto and Brenda about helping me provide the nutritional basis and peer-reviewed research showing how the Raw Food Revolution Diet could not only help people lose weight and feel better in the short term, but help them become healthier for life, I experienced a bit of professional skepticism. They had not yet personally experienced an entirely raw diet and had encountered little peer-reviewed nutritional data that could validate what I had experienced and observed. Both of these highly respected women were willing to look into the subject. After a year of careful research, they came to the conclusion that the Raw Food Revolution Diet can indeed deliver what so many people have experienced firsthand. This is a way of eating that allows people to feast, lose weight, gain energy, and feel younger.

It's more than a diet—it's a lifestyle that has the power to fuel a revolution! If you're tired of looking in the mirror and seeing the person staring back at you, isn't it time you took control of your life and joined the raw diet revolution?

Brenda: *Widening the Circle of Compassion*

Back in high school, I was a nutrition nut, so it was no surprise to anyone when I choose human nutrition as my major in university. Following my internship in 1983, I accepted a position as a community nutritionist in northern Ontario. Most of what I taught was based on the Nutrition Recommendations for Canadians and Canada's Food Guide, which included meat and fish as well as dairy products. Although I was immersed in the world of "healthful" omnivorous diets, I was not entirely committed. I was intrigued by vegetarianism but had only ever met one real live vegetarian in my life: my eighth-grade science teacher. He was a hippie of sorts, and people thought rather ill of him for forcing a vegetarian lifestyle on his family. During my university studies, we learned two things about vegetarian diets: vegetarian diets that include eggs and dairy products (lacto-ovo) are risky, especially for children and pregnant or lactating women, and vegan diets, which are based completely on plant foods, are downright dangerous. In spite of it all, I found myself slowly shifting toward a plant-based diet.

Then, without any warning, the unthinkable happened. A hunter's carefully chosen words pushed me over the edge (although I don't think that was his intention). This longtime friend called to see if he could stop by for coffee on his way deer hunting. After dispensing with the usual trivialities, I asked him how he could justify pulling the trigger on such a beautiful animal. I pointed out that it wasn't fair—the deer had no defense against his bullet. I asked him if it made him feel like more of a man to shoot a defenseless creature. His response changed the course of my life. He said, "You have no right to criticize me. Just because you don't have the guts to pull the trigger does not mean you are not responsible for the trigger being pulled every time you buy a piece of meat in the grocery store. You are simply paying someone to do the dirty work for you. At least the deer I eat has had a life. I doubt very much you can say the same for the animals sitting on your plate." I was silenced, because I knew deep down inside that he was absolutely right. At that moment I vowed to take responsibility for the food I was purchasing and learn about the lives of the animals I was eating. What I discovered sickened me to the point that I knew I would never eat another piece of flesh as long as I lived.

As you might appreciate, I faced some interesting personal and professional challenges. First, my family—how would they react? My children were one and four years old. My husband grew up in northern Ontario—not exactly a bastion of vegetarianism. Almost all of his best friends were hunters. To my amazement, when I asked him if he would be willing to make the switch with me, he said, "I thought you'd never ask." He was a committed environmentalist and was happy to do just about anything that he believed would lessen his impact on the planet.

Because the dietetic profession is so influenced by the meat and dairy industries, I could not even imagine being a vegetarian dietitian. But I came to the conclusion that our profession was due for a change, and it would most likely be the result of a force from within. It has been a joy and a privilege to witness the progressive changes in the fields of nutrition and dietetics, and it is especially encouraging to see so many talented young vegans making this their chosen profession.

Working on this book has added a whole new dimension to my raw evolution. When I began, my diet was about 50% raw. Today it is closer to 80% raw and continuing to rise as I fall in love with the recipes in this book. Initially, I was a little apprehensive about buying new kitchen tools and learning how to use them, and exploring a world that challenges my science-based thinking. While some raw food can be a lot of work to prepare, it doesn't all have to be, and it gets easier with practice. I have been surprised and impressed at how easy it was to switch from roasted almonds to soaked and dehydrated almonds, from store-bought crackers to raw flax crackers, and from cooked soups to delightful raw soups. One of the great perks is the reduction in waste—needless to say, raw foods require minimal packaging and little gas or electricity to prepare. Best of all, eating a raw diet opened a whole new world of fabulous culinary experiences and many exciting health benefits. For me, the most notice-able benefit was to my energy level. I don't have the afternoon slumps I used to have. I run faster and need less sleep. It is quite wonderful.

At the time of this writing, I'm in my late forties and Cherie and Vesanto are in their sixties. I am absolutely inspired by them. Think about what the average 60-year-old North American woman looks and feels like. Most are overweight and have high blood pressure, high cholesterol, diabetes, or arthritis, or a combination of these ailments. The usual response to such a health crisis is medications or surgery. Unfortunately, there are no medications and no surgeries that have ever or will ever cure lifestyle-induced diseases. The only thing that will ever reverse them are positive lifestyle choices. Making healthful choices is no sacrifice at all; it is a privilege to be cherished. Health is the real ticket to freedom.

Vesanto: *My Gourmet Raw Weight-Loss Adventure*

Prior to writing this raw book, I had seven very popular food and nutrition books to my credit, books that are now in 14 countries and 4 languages. What was the outcome of all that effort? Fame? Yes, a little. Speaking invitations? These took me from Hawaii to Barcelona, and many places in between. What else? All those hours sitting at the computer, inter-spersed with breaks for recipe testing, resulted in . . . fat. Yes, about 20 extra pounds.

I decided it was time to lighten up. What would be the solution?

I attempted a raw diet on my own for a few weeks. With fruit salad for breakfast, green salad for lunch, and another big salad for supper, I did lose a few pounds. But it became so boring that my old habits crept in. Another weight-loss plan was derailed.

The raw solution continued to hold appeal. I wanted to feel slim, light, and somewhat more youthful. Drawn on by my curiosity, I enrolled at the renowned Living Light Culinary Arts Institute in Fort Bragg, California, midway between San Francisco and the California-Oregon border.

I had signed up for several courses, knowing that for a shift in dietary habits to take hold, I would require a few weeks of immersion. My first course consisted of a weekend of demos by expert chefs, followed by sampling—or, to be accurate, by feasting. The food that was created far surpassed what I had envisioned. During the following week, I had hands-on experience in creating tasty, raw cuisine where we learned to combine flavors and develop our own recipes. It was becoming deliciously clear that a mainly or entirely raw diet wouldn't be so bad after all.

To get the most out of this experience, I decided to keep my diet as raw as I could comfortably manage. It wasn't all smooth sailing. On occasional afternoons, I experienced drops in blood sugar. Thinking back, though, I realized that I *always* have midafternoon dips in energy. Before, I had relied on fat- and sugar-laden snacks and sweet tea to boost my energy. Here we had the opportunity to experiment broadly and see what would be our most effective energy boosters: a green drink, selections from an abundant bowl of fruit, raw veggies, or occasionally a slice of gourmet fruit pie or a raw cookie made of nuts and dried fruit.

In this supportive environment, eating 100% raw turned out to be entirely achievable. An early observation was that I needed less sleep. I slept deeply and awakened feeling completely refreshed 30–60 minutes earlier than usual. It's common knowledge that heavy foods take energy to digest, so it's not surprising that increased vigor and energy is a frequent experience of raw food enthusiasts. I was starting to feel lighter and discovered extra space inside my waistband.

In accordance with my highest hopes, the pounds did melt away. After an initial weekend loss of four pounds, I shed between one and three pounds a week. Even after leaving Living Light this continued, as long as I retained my focus on raw plant foods. I could eat delicious salad dressings, savory nut or seed pâtés, and creamy avocado soups, though I found that I had to put reasonable limits on these higher-fat foods. My plate could be piled high with colorful veggies, and still there was room for the occasional wedge of raw chocolate cake or fruit torte. I felt full; I felt satisfied.

As a dietitian, I was fascinated with the nutritional adequacy of the foods I ate. With my vegan diet, I had been used to a fairly high protein intake. It turned out that a day's raw menu could entirely meet recommendations for protein, minerals, omega-3 fatty acids, and vitamins, with a supplementary source of vitamin B_{12}. (For examples of raw menus that meet all the recommended nutrient intakes, see pages 92–100.)

Those of us who are challenged by weight management tend to have specific cravings that are our downfall. A diet centered on raw plant foods automatically gets us past these downfalls. Fruits provide a sweet treat.

Veggie choices are filling yet they contain few calories. Mineral-rich seeds and nuts can be made into the most delectable replacements for favorite foods.

I discovered that a raw diet can be superbly simple. In its raw form, corn on the cob now has more appeal than cooked. While traveling through Belgium and wandering around Paris, I discovered the joys of filling my day pack with pea pods and cherry tomatoes.

I'm heading into this next stage of my life in fine form. In fact, my medical doctor regularly sends clients to me for nutrition counseling. I enjoy a vegan diet that is entirely raw on some days and mainly raw on others. At the age of 65, I am in excellent health and annually take part in a triathlon. With the combination of regular weight-bearing exercise and care taken to meet recommended calcium and vitamin D intakes, my bone density has actually increased slightly in the last few years—no small feat at this age!

Should you have the opportunity to attend the Living Light Culinary Arts Institute, you'll be well rewarded. If you wish to lighten up your body and spirit, this is the place for your transformation.

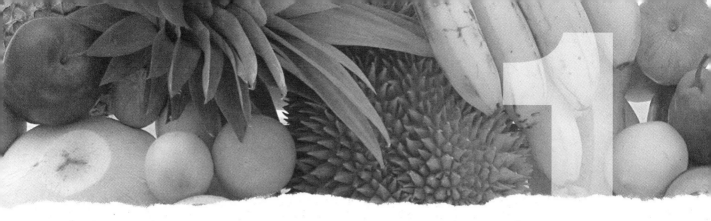

take the first step
toward vibrant living

Our health is a reflection of the way we experience life. The SAD (an acronym for Standard American Diet) truth is that most people do not know what it means to live a healthy, vibrant life. Many people think they are healthy because they have no visible symptoms of illness, but the best way to measure health is to look at the amount of vitality and enthusiasm one has for life. Today, millions of people are literally sick and tired from living fast, eating fast, and eating fast foods that are completely devoid of the most important ingredient of all: love! Most of these fast foods are cooked, refined, often fried, and toxic to our bodies. Foods are eaten on the go or in front of the TV, without awareness or appreciation for the nourishment they provide. The increasing number of people who are sick, depressed, and walking around in a lowered state of consciousness is a telling story of how we live our lives.

Taking care of yourself is the best insurance you have for a life of joy and good health. Health insurance, which is actually disease and accident insurance, cannot provide what a good lifestyle can offer in terms of well-being. And no amount of so-called health insurance can provide the sense of joy and well-being that a health-promoting lifestyle can.

THE OBESITY BATTLE—HOW DID WE GET HERE?

Americans have more choices when it comes to food than anyone else on the planet. While we are constantly seduced by hot fudge sundaes, double cheeseburgers, stuffed-crust pizza, and deep-fried doughnuts, we are expected to be as lean as the models that grace the covers of fashion magazines. How many people have the willpower to resist temptation time and time again? A very small minority, it would seem. In 2005, approximately two-thirds of the American adult population was classified as overweight or obese, with about one-third fitting into the overweight category and the other third being obese. The harsh reality is that fewer than one-third of Americans have healthy body weights. A July 2007 study from the Johns Hopkins Bloomberg School of Public Health estimated that, at the current rate of growth, 75% of American adults and almost 25% of American children will be overweight or obese by 2015. Some experts go so far as to suggest that, at our current rate of expansion, almost every one of us will be fat by the year 2025.

This is no minor inconvenience. Overweight and obesity come with a hefty price tag—$100 billion a year in medical bills and more than 400,000 premature deaths each year. Excess body fat causes unwanted changes to the basic functioning of the human body, adversely affecting blood pressure, cholesterol, triglycerides, respiration, fertility, skin and joint health, hormones, and insulin action. Such changes significantly increase the risk for debilitating and often fatal health conditions, including the following:

- cancer
- gallbladder disease
- gout
- heart disease and stroke
- kidney disease
- osteoarthritis
- sleep apnea
- type 2 diabetes

To add insult to injury, a recent report found that being obese effectively ages a person by 20 years (in terms of physical health). That puts an obese 30-year-old in the same risk group as a normal-weight 50-year-old for developing serious medical problems.

Being overweight or obese is not something many of us aspire to. In fact, given the choice, very few of us would choose to be overweight or obese. So why are so many people affected?

There is little doubt that too much food and too little exercise are technically responsible for the North American overweight and obesity epidemic. However, for most individuals, overweight and obesity are the result of a complex interplay of many factors: physical, environmental, and emotional.

Physical Factors

While we may all be created equal, we are not all the same. It seems that certain people require more physical activity and fewer calories to maintain a healthy body weight than their peers. This is sometimes referred to as a slow metabolism. In the face of food abundance and a sedentary lifestyle, such people are at greater risk for overweight, obesity, and chronic disease. Extremely low-calorie diets serve only to make matters worse, as they signal the body to move into conservation mode, further slowing metabolism. Yet while a slow metabolism is a reality for some people, many others mistakenly believe that the blame for their problem rests here. Obesity researchers have found that, in truth, overweight and obese people commonly consume double the number of calories that they believe they are eating. For most people, overeating trumps a slow metabolism when it comes to weight gain.

Less commonly, overweight and obesity are triggered by medications or endocrine disorders such as hypothyroidism (an underactive thyroid reduces metabolic rate). While such causes are relatively rare, they do occur and can make it extremely difficult to succeed at weight loss.

Another factor that is just beginning to emerge as a major player is appetite control. When our appetite control center is overwhelmed, desensitized, or otherwise impaired, this system can be thrown off balance, resulting in weight gain. While we are just beginning to understand the workings of this system, it appears that many dietary factors can have an impact. For example, diets rich in fat, refined sugars (especially refined high-fructose products), and refined starches appear to have a negative effect.

Environmental Factors

Our culture has established the perfect environment for weight gain. Food is abundant and accessible at home, at work, and everywhere in between. Food is at the center of our social gatherings, from birth to death. All too often, indulging means a heaping plate of nutritionally depleted, fat-and-sugar-laden processed food. To make matters worse, portion sizes, like our waistbands, keep expanding. In the 1960s, a family-sized soft drink bottle was 26 ounces (810 mL), allowing for four servings, each 6.5 ounces (195 mL). Today, in many restaurants and theaters, a "small" serving of soda is 16–20 ounces (500–620 mL). Muffins and bagels have doubled in size since the 1970s, and portion sizes of many entrées have also swelled. Consumers are lured by supersizing—the offer of much more food for just a little extra money. The bargains are irresistible. For a mere 25–50% more money, you can often receive 100–300% more food. The problem is that when we are served larger portions, we eat more. It's human nature.

In addition, most of us have sedentary jobs, and in our spare time we watch television, play video games, or surf the Net. Every possible convenience has been developed to help save us time and energy. In this environment, staying slim seems a greater challenge than becoming overweight or obese.

the appetite control center

The appetite control center is housed in a part of the brain called the hypothalamus. There are many hormones that affect it; here are the most important ones:

Ghrelin stimulates appetite. It's released when the stomach is empty, and its release stops when we eat. Carbohydrates and protein appear to suppress this appetite-stimulating hormone more than fat does, which seems to be one of the reasons that high-fat diets promote weight gain.

Leptin, *insulin*, and *amylin* work together to reduce appetite. Both leptin and insulin dampen appetite by inhibiting neurons in the appetite control center that stimulate appetite, and by stimulating neurons that depress appetite. Leptin is released from fat tissue, and as the amount of body fat grows, leptin levels also increase. It would be logical to assume this would work to the advantage of people who are obese, as leptin reduces appetite. However, research suggests that the appetite control center becomes resistant to leptin when levels are unusually high over time. Consequently, leptin would be less efficient at suppressing hunger. Weight loss helps to reduce body fat and leptin secretion; it also helps to restore leptin sensitivity.

The story for insulin is strikingly similar. Insulin is released by the pancreas. As body fat increases, the risk of insulin resistance also increases (a condition in which the body fails to use insulin properly). The pancreas pumps out even more insulin in an effort to compensate. Not surprisingly, when the body becomes resistant to insulin, the appetite control center also becomes resistant to insulin. With increasing weight gain, a vicious cycle is set in motion: appetite control is lost, energy expenditure slows down, and eating increases. As is the case with leptin, weight loss helps to decrease insulin secretion and restore insulin sensitivity.

Amylin is secreted along with insulin from the pancreas. This hormone works together with insulin to slow emptying of the stomach. Amylin reduces hunger and helps to control body weight.

All in all, overweight and obesity seem to upset the delicate balance of appetite-control hormones. Fortunately, with a healthful lifestyle and weight loss, this balance can be restored.

Emotional Factors

For many people, weight gain has as much to do with managing life's challenges and social pressures as it does with overeating and underactivity. Difficult interactions, disappointment, embarrassment, stress, or hardship all seem to be eased by food, even when we're not hungry. Successes, victories, and other joyous moments also seem to provide reasons to reward oneself with favorite foods. Eating in response to emotions rather than physical hunger is known as emotional eating.

For some people, excess body weight is used as a shield to protect against the pain associated with life and love. Being obese means being safe—it allows for an escape from situations that could be too difficult to face. Of course, these "advantages" are deceiving, as they generally serve only to hide the true self, and they come at an enormous cost to both physical and emotional well-being.

In its most severe form, emotional eating can lead to eating disorders such as compulsive overeating, or binge-eating disorder, where very large quantities of food are consumed. Compulsive-overeating disorder is related to anorexia nervosa and bulimia nervosa, but it doesn't involve food restriction or purging after gorging—so it often results in obesity. Most people are surprised to learn that compulsive overeating is the most common type of eating disorder in America. It affects an estimated 25 million people—more than double the estimated 12 million suffering from anorexia nervosa and bulimia nervosa combined.

WINNING THE BATTLE OF THE BULGE: A PLAN FOR LIFE

At any one time, approximately 20–40% of the American population is actively attempting to lose weight. Weight-loss diets are generally designed to produce a calorie deficit, or to ensure that you take in fewer calories than you burn, so you will lose weight. Most succeed in this task. When it comes to weight loss, whether you eat grapefruits, cabbage soup, or bacon and eggs matters far less than the number of calories you consume. So, all sorts of food combinations can do the trick, as long as they leave you with a calorie deficit.

Even though most diets succeed in producing weight loss, the problem is, they end. When they do, the weight creeps back on. About 95% of all weight-loss diets are utter failures in the long term. In many cases, the deprivation causes your body to move into conservation mode, slowing your metabolism. You not only regain the lost weight, you may end up gaining additional pounds as well. *In order to achieve a lifelong healthful weight, you need lifelong healthful eating and exercise habits. There is no going back to your former diet and lifestyle—ever.*

From the perspective of the consumer, the fatal flaw of the weight-loss industry is that their primary focus is earning a profit, not permanent weight loss. Return customers are part of the game plan. The weight-loss industry has great expertise in telling their customers what they want to hear: "Lose all the weight you want for only $30"; "Melt fat while you sleep"; "Speed your metabolism and drop pounds without dieting." So what's the answer? Stop buying into hype and start buying into health. The following three simple steps will put you on a path that moves your focus beyond thin.

Step #1: Make great health, energy, and vitality your goals.

Dump the dieter's mentality of thinness at all costs. It is not worth the risk. Remember, thinness can be the reward for healthful living or the curse of illness or substance abuse. It can be achieved by eating greens or undergoing chemotherapy. Without health, energy, and vitality, a lean body loses its luster.

The first and most critical step to permanently overcoming overweight and obesity is to redirect your focus from thinness to health. This is no small feat, particularly in Western culture. Begin by looking at food as the raw materials with which you will rebuild your body. Resist the urge to select food on the basis of its consequences for your body weight. Instead, select food on the basis of its ability to nourish and protect your body. Before you bite into that sugar-free "diet" cookie, ask yourself if white flour, partially hydrogenated vegetable oils, and artificial sweeteners are the materials with which you'd like to build your brain cells. Hopefully the very thought will leave a bad taste in your mouth. Perhaps an apple would be more appealing.

Resist the temptation to measure your success on the basis of the bathroom scale. While it's okay to weigh yourself on occasion, daily weigh-ins are a lesson in frustration. Focus instead on how you feel. Know that as your health, energy, and vitality are restored, your weight will gradually adjust to a point that is ideal for your body. Remember, a healthy body weight is a natural consequence of a health-promoting lifestyle.

Step #2: Think positively.

What are your greatest dreams for body, mind, and spirit? How close to achieving them could you be in a month, a year, or five years? Hold on to those dreams. No matter how far away you are, know that every tiny step you take toward your ultimate goal is worth celebrating. Remember, life is not a competition, and it is not about being perfect. It is far more important that you have found a path that supports your physical, emotional, and spiritual well-being than how far you have come along the path.

Push out any negative thoughts with positive affirmations. Remind yourself that you will achieve what you have set your mind to achieve, that you will move forward toward your goals, and that there is nothing anyone can do to extinguish your enthusiasm.

As you work to develop positive habits, be prepared for stumbling blocks and resistance. Don't beat yourself up when things don't go according to plan. Instead, use each disappointment as a guide to making better choices next time.

Step #3: Build healthful habits.

Break old, destructive diet and lifestyle patterns. Do you recall the story about a wise teacher who taught her students about the power of bad habits with a spool of thread? She asked a student to hold his wrists together and she wound the thread around just once. Then she asked him if he could break the thread. He did so easily. She explained to her class that this illustrates the power of doing something once. Then she took the thread and wound it around the student's wrists many times. Once again she asked him if he could break the thread. No matter how hard he tried, the thread was too strong to be broken. She explained to her class that this illustrates the power of doing something repeatedly.

When we do something often enough, it gets so integrated into our daily lives that it becomes automatic. We call these kinds of responses habits. When they have negative consequences for our health and general well-being, they are called bad habits. Bad habits don't tend to vanish spontaneously. Generally, breaking a bad habit takes determination and perseverance.

The first critical step in breaking a bad habit is to get acquainted with the habit. Why has it been so successful in seducing you? What makes it so difficult to let it go? Become intimately aware of the reality of your behavior and erase the fantasy that has served as its justification. You must see the habit for what it really is—your enemy in life and health.

Next, carefully construct a game plan. The plan must involve more than simply breaking the bad habit. It must replace the bad habit with something of value to your life and health—a *good* habit. To make your plan foolproof, be sure to set it up so you are surrounded by a strong support system.

WHAT IS A HEALTHY BODY WEIGHT?

There is no one "ideal" weight for a person of a particular height because our healthiest weight depends on our bone structure, muscle mass, body fat, and general body build. However, the definitions that follow help determine if a person is overweight or obese:

- Overweight—at least 10% above a healthy body weight (for most people that is about 10–30 pounds over their healthy body weight)
- Obese—at least 20% above a healthy body weight (for most people that is 30 pounds or more above their healthy body weight)

The very best way to know if you are within a healthy weight range is to determine how much of your body weight is fat. A body fat level greater

body mass index

BMI is recommended for people age 20–65, but it does not factor in muscle mass. Very muscular people will have a high BMI but could have a very low percentage of body fat; thus they would appear overweight according to the BMI, even though they are actually very lean. Very short people (under 5 feet/1.5 meters tall) may have a higher BMI than would be expected relative to their size. BMI is not useful for pregnant women or those over the age of 65.

A BMI of 18.5–24.9 is considered in the healthy weight range. Those with a BMI below 18.5 are considered underweight and at increased health risk. A BMI of 25–29.9 is considered overweight. Obesity is generally defined as a BMI of 30 or greater; severe obesity is 35 or greater, and morbid or extreme obesity is 40 or greater. *Research suggests that those with a BMI of 19–22 enjoy the greatest longevity.*

than 17% in men and 27% in women indicates overweight, while a body fat level of greater than 25% in men and 31% in women indicates obesity.

Getting accurate body fat measurements can be a challenge. The most widely used method of determining body fatness is called body mass index (BMI). To find your BMI, plot your height and weight on table 1.

WHAT IS YOUR BODY SHAPE?

Knowing body shape can help to eliminate some of the inconsistencies associated with BMI. If you carry the bulk of your weight above your hips (mainly in your abdomen), you have an apple shape. If you are an apple shape, weight gain tends to go directly to your stomach. This body shape is more common in men than women.

If excess weight is carried in your extremities (your hips, thighs, and buttocks), you are said to have a pear shape. People who are pear shaped generally have larger hips than waist. This body shape is more common in women.

You can also determine whether you have an apple or pear shape by calculating your waist-to-hip ratio. Simply take a measurement of your waist and hips and divide the waist measurement by the hip measurement. A ratio of 0.80 or less for women and 0.90 or less for men is considered a pear shape. If you are overweight or obese, having an apple shape puts you at much higher risk for heart disease, type 2 diabetes, hypertension, and several types of cancer. For those who naturally become apple shaped

what is a healthy body weight?

TABLE 1 Body Mass Index (BMI)

Ht (in)	60	61	62	63	64	65	66	67	68	69	70	71	72	73	74	75
BMI	**Body Weight (pounds)**															
17	87	90	93	96	99	102	105	108	111	115	118	121	125	129	132	135
18	92	95	98	101	106	108	111	114	118	122	125	128	132	136	140	143
19	97	100	104	107	110	114	118	121	125	128	132	136	140	144	148	152
20	102	106	109	113	116	120	124	127	131	135	139	143	147	151	155	160
21	107	111	115	118	122	126	130	134	138	142	146	150	154	159	163	168
22	112	116	120	124	128	132	136	140	144	149	153	157	162	166	171	176
23	118	122	126	130	134	138	142	146	151	155	160	165	169	174	179	184
24	123	127	131	135	140	144	148	153	158	162	167	172	177	182	186	192
25	128	132	136	141	145	150	155	159	164	169	174	179	184	189	194	200
26	133	137	141	146	151	156	161	166	171	176	181	186	191	197	202	208
27	138	143	146	152	157	162	167	172	177	182	188	193	199	204	210	216
28	143	148	152	158	163	168	173	178	184	189	195	200	206	212	218	224
29	148	153	158	163	169	174	179	185	190	196	202	208	213	219	225	232
30	153	158	164	169	174	180	186	191	197	203	209	215	221	227	233	241
31	158	164	169	175	180	186	192	198	203	209	216	222	228	235	241	248
32	163	169	175	180	186	192	198	204	210	216	222	228	235	242	249	256
33	168	174	180	186	192	198	204	211	216	223	229	236	242	250	256	264
34	174	180	186	191	197	204	210	217	223	230	236	243	250	257	264	272
35	179	185	191	197	204	210	216	223	230	236	243	250	258	265	272	279
36	184	190	196	203	209	215	223	229	236	243	250	257	265	272	280	286
37	189	195	201	208	215	221	229	235	243	250	257	264	272	280	287	294
38	194	201	206	214	221	227	235	242	249	257	264	271	279	288	295	302
39	199	206	212	220	227	233	241	248	256	263	271	278	287	295	303	310
40	204	211	218	225	232	239	247	254	262	270	278	285	294	303	311	318

UNDERSTANDING YOUR BMI

BMI < 18.5: May indicate underweight

BMI 18.5–24.9: Healthy weight for most people

BMI 25–29.9: Indicates overweight

BMI ≥ 30: Indicates obesity

BMI ≥ 35: Indicates severe obesity

BMI ≥ 40: Indicates extreme or morbid obesity

with weight gain, it is critically important that a healthy body weight be maintained.

Finally, a waist measurement of over 32 inches (81 cm) for women and 37 inches (94 cm) for men suggests that you should try to avoid gaining any weight. A measurement of 35 inches (89 cm) for women and 40 inches (102 cm) for men indicates overweight and that health improvements could be expected with weight loss.

THE RAW FOOD REVOLUTION DIET SOLUTION

Taking the first step toward vibrant living is easy—simply add more raw plant-based foods to your diet. It's a profound way of taking responsibility for your own well-being and taking the road to conscious, joyful living. The results are a trimmer body, better health, more energy, more enjoyment of the foods you eat, and more appreciation of the simpler things in life. This back-to-nature approach to eating provides more life to our bodies, minds, and spirits, and enables us to appreciate the gift of being fully alive.

People are often surprised that when they begin the Raw Food Revolution Diet they find greater enjoyment in eating than they did on their previous SAD diet. This depth of satisfaction is not only physical— it is mental and spiritual as well. Eating more raw food increases one's health and encourages a mindful appreciation of life and a greater connection with nature. This does not mean that eating cooked food is bad, only that the more we replace cooked food with raw food in our diets, the more vitality, clarity of mind, and presence of being we experience. Another beneficial side effect is it enables us to establish our natural body weight, which, for most people, means losing weight.

Eating raw food does not mean giving up the ecstatic pleasure of food. On the contrary, raw foods, prepared consciously, are even more pleasing. When we prepare food in a state of appreciation, love is transferred through the food to us. Simple, delicious, raw food prepared with loving consciousness leaves us feeling lighter and freer in all aspects of our being. Perhaps there is another part of us besides the physical body that requires nourishment and cannot be measured by scientists.

Many people who transition to the Raw Food Revolution Diet find that they require much less sleep and feel better immediately. Others experience rapid detoxification, because raw food can stimulate cleansing of both the physical and emotional bodies. Therefore, unless you are gravely ill (in which case we propose that you consult your medical doctor), try increasing the amount of raw food in your diet gradually, over time, to avoid cleansing reactions such as headaches, dermatitis, lethargy, stomachaches, gas, and emotional outbursts. Make your transition more enjoyable by listening to your body and increasing the amount of raw food in your diet moderately and gently.

Many people think it's difficult or complicated to get started on a raw food diet, that it takes a long time to prepare the food and requires special equipment. The truth is it can be as simple as peeling a banana or as complicated as making Bananas! I Scream (page 220) with Fruit Coulis (page 222). They are both good—it's up to you how much time you want to spend in the kitchen. A simple smoothie or blended soup can be easy to prepare and still be delicious and totally satisfying. Then again, sometimes you may want to prepare something more complex, like raw veggie burgers with all the trimmings. Most of the comfort foods you now enjoy can be prepared without cooking if you set up your kitchen to support a new way of preparing food so it will taste delicious and nourish you on all levels.

RAW FOOD DIETS: ARE THEY ALL THE SAME?

When we speak of a raw food diet, we are proposing it not only as a 21-day weight-loss regimen; we also propose it as a way of life that will help you balance your weight—once and for all—gain more energy, feel younger and more vibrant, and best of all, do it without counting calories or giving up the satisfaction of delicious food.

There are many health professionals who disagree on the "perfect" raw food diet, but there are some things that almost all the experts in the field of raw nutrition agree on: animal products should be eliminated. There is a very small segment of raw food eaters who consume raw meat, but they are rare (no pun intended). Most raw food enthusiasts (also called raw fooders or raw foodists) choose ripe, raw, organic, high-water-content, seasonal fruits and vegetables; some nuts and seeds; pure (chlorine- and fluoride-free) water; and lots of dark leafy greens. Grains, beans, and legumes, if eaten, are sprouted. Gluten-free or low-gluten grains (such as amaranth and quinoa) are the ones most often recommended for those who choose to eat grains.

Raw food enthusiasts typically say no to highly processed foods like wheat products (pasta, bread, and pastries), processed sugars (especially white sugar), deep-fried foods, hard liquor, and products containing additives and preservatives.

Some of this may seem extreme, but while you follow the eating plan in this book, keep an open mind and just eat as much raw food as you feel comfortable doing. Even adding an extra salad each day to a cooked diet can make a big difference.

raw food standards

During the International Living Food Summit held at the Hippocrates Health Institute in West Palm Beach, Florida, on January 14, 2006, living food movement leaders from eight countries (with a combined total of 411 years following this lifestyle) agreed on the following standards.

THE OPTIMUM DIET FOR HEALTH AND LONGEVITY

- vegan (no animal products of any kind, cooked or raw)
- organic
- whole foods
- high in nutrition (such as vitamins, antioxidants, and phytonutrients)
- contains a significant amount of minerals
- contains a significant quantity of highly nutritious green foods
- contains adequate complete protein from plant sources
- contains a large proportion of high-water-content foods
- provides excellent hydration
- includes raw vegetable juices
- contains all essential fatty acids, including omega-3 fatty acids from naturally occurring plant sources
- is at least 80% raw (with the remainder of the diet vegan, whole food, and organic)
- has moderate yet adequate calories
- contains only low to moderate sugar, exclusively from whole food sources (fruitarianism is strongly discouraged)
- is nutritionally optimal for both detoxification and rebuilding

IT WAS ALSO AGREED THAT

- supplementation with vitamin B_{12} is advised;
- the addition of whole food supplements is advised;
- this way of eating can be further optimized by tailoring it based on individual needs (within the principles stated);
- benefits derived by following these principles are proportional to how well they are followed;
- we will remain open-minded, and this information will be updated and expanded upon, if necessary, as new research becomes available;
- diet is a critical piece of a healthy lifestyle, yet not the entire picture.

A full-spectrum, health-supporting lifestyle is encouraged. This includes physical exercise, exposure to sunshine, and maintaining good psychological health. Avoiding environmental toxins and toxic products is essential. Paramount is pure water (for consumption and bathing) and the use of natural-fiber clothing and nontoxic personal care products. Healthful options in home furnishings, building materials, and related items should also be considered.

All leaders agree that the main objective of eating an optimal diet in accordance with the Raw Food Standards is to promote health and prevent and minimize disease.

WHAT IS FOOD COMBINING?

Food combining is a popular adjunct to many raw diets. It's based on the theory that different food groups require different digestion times. According to food-combining principles, digestion is made easier if we don't eat foods simultaneously that require different amounts of time to break down. Food combining guidelines state that

- proteins take longer to digest than starches;
- concentrated proteins, such as nuts, meat, and dairy products, can be eaten with green leafy vegetables but interfere with good digestion when combined with starchy vegetables, such as potatoes, root vegetables, and grains;
- protein should never be eaten with fruit;
- fruits should be eaten alone, as they digest more quickly than other foods.

The purpose of proper food combining is to make it easy for our bodies to digest and assimilate our meals. According to food-combining principles, each food belongs in four to nine categories (food-combining experts differ on the number of categories, so you will likely encounter some varying opinions). Each category is said to combine well or poorly with foods in other categories. For instance, fats do not combine well with fruits or starches, protein does not combine well with starches, fruits do not combine well with anything other than leafy greens, and melons do not combine well with any other foods. Food-combining "rules" are complicated and difficult to adhere to, especially for those of us who enjoy prepared food combinations, such as raw oatmeal with bananas or a raw fruit pie with a grain or nut crust. Complicating these principles even more is the fact that every vegetable, seed, fruit, and other raw food in its natural form is a combination of protein, fat, and carbohydrate.

Even though there are many people in the raw food community teaching hard-and-fast rules about the theory of food combining, there is no scientific evidence to date to support it. Food combining has been advocated since the early 1900s, adopted by early natural hygienists and other raw food advocates such as Ann Wigmore, and is still being taught by raw food teachers today.

Rick and Karin Dina, who are strong advocates of the raw food lifestyle and have a combined 33 years of living, studying, and teaching raw food nutrition, tell us that since the time food combining was theorized, physiologists have learned that the stomach is always acid and the small intestine is always alkaline, no matter what foods are eaten. When a plant food that contains mostly carbohydrates is consumed, digestion starts with the salivary amylase in the mouth, then moves on to the acidic environment of the stomach, and continues in the small intestine. When a food high in protein is eaten, digestion takes place primarily in the stomach due to the acidity there. Food combining, as it is taught by many proponents, suggests that if you eat a protein and starch together, the body wears itself out producing both alkaline and acidic digestive juices, which end up cancelling each other out and impairing digestion, and that, according to the Dinas, is simply not true.

Modern, scientifically oriented natural hygiene doctors believe that food combining can be useful to the extent that it helps people to simplify their meals, therefore allowing them greater likelihood of eating within their digestive capacity and improving their digestion. But for most people this may not be a major issue of concern.

According to the Dinas, even though it has not been scientifically proven, the one principle of food combining that makes sense is to avoid eating fruit and heavier food at the same time. Many people report improved digestion when fresh fruit is eaten apart from other foods or at the beginning of the meal. While many people tolerate combining fruits with other foods, it is important to listen to your body and do what works best for you. It is worth noting that eating vitamin C–rich fruits with other foods can have advantages for anyone on a plant-based diet because they help to increase the absorption of iron in other foods (see page 58).

Certainly, if you are experiencing symptoms of bloating, gas, or indigestion, keep a journal of your eating habits and see if there are certain foods or combinations of foods that appear to cause difficulty. Other factors may also contribute to indigestion, not the least of which are stress and negative emotions while eating.

The bottom line is there's no scientific backing for the concept of food combining. If you're just learning a new way of eating, there are far more important issues to be concerned with, and the restrictions of food combining can often be too burdensome. More important than any science, be aware that indigestion might be improved by avoiding certain food combinations.

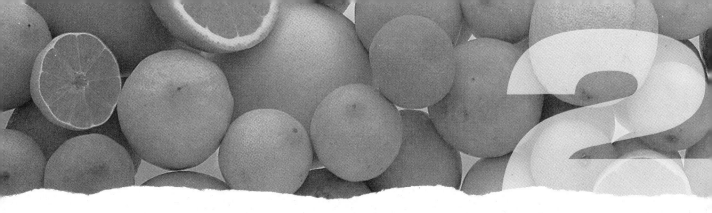

achieve permanent weight loss with the Raw Food Revolution Diet

Now that you have some background on the Raw Food Revolution Diet, let's talk about why it's so easy to lose weight and keep it off by going raw.

RAW FOOD: WEAPONS OF MASS REDUCTION

While there are many things we can do to improve our food choices, there are few that are more powerful and effective than incorporating more whole, raw plant foods into our diets. When we choose more raw foods, we also choose fewer foods that are at the root of our obesity epidemic. These are foods that call out to us. It is no mere coincidence that they are extraordinarily satisfying. Neal Barnard, MD, sums it up well in his book *Breaking the Food Seduction*:

> What if someone invented a chemical that could trigger the brain's pleasure circuits—a chemical that did not make you stronger, help you reproduce, or assist you in any other way—but still gave your brain a feeling so warm and pleasant that you would want to repeat it over and over? Well, someone did. Heroin, cocaine, alcohol, nicotine, and, in fact, all recreational drugs work on the brain's pleasure center, triggering a greatly exaggerated dopamine response.
>
> Someone also invented chocolate bars, wedges of cheese, cookies, and doughnuts. All of these foods are capable of stimulating precisely the same part of the brain that responds to heroin. And that is why they can be addicting. The fact is, we've been a bit too clever for our own good, refining food products to the point where they provide all the pleasure and very little of the nutrition we need.

While you may feel very apprehensive about removing these foods from your diet, it's absolutely amazing what happens when you replace these high-fat, high-sugar foods with others that promote health and healing. Your body restores its balance and you begin to feel a freedom that is inexplicable. When your body is nourished with everything you need for optimal health and well-being, you feel satisfied; there is no sense of deprivation. Your body is better able to handle the occasional junk food, but you are far less likely to crave it.

Plans for Success

As you prepare for your raw food adventure, you'll notice that you have a decision to make regarding your initiation. The Raw Food Revolution Diet offers a three-week Fast Track plan; although it is optional, we highly recommend it. The following information will help you determine whether or not to begin with the Fast Track.

The Fast Track is a three-week, intensive, 100% raw diet plan that serves to "rewire" your system, including your taste buds. It provides a cleansing of sorts. Beginning on the Fast Track will result in significant health changes in a relatively short period of time. Initial weight loss with this plan will be more dramatic than if you begin with the Raw Food Revolution Diet, although both options are highly effective long term. The Fast Track requires a greater degree of personal commitment in terms of time and energy. The focus is strictly on you for three full weeks.

Cut back on foods you that keep you hooked, such as white sugar, cooked starches, fried foods, salty condiments, chocolate, coffee, and alcohol.

The Raw Food Revolution Diet is a long-term plan that will help you to attain and maintain a healthy weight for life. It allows for a greater variety of food than is recommended on the Fast Track, and some cooked food is permitted. The Raw Food Revolution Diet provides 80% or more of calories from raw food and up to 20% of calories from cooked food. It is both manageable and appealing.

How do you know whether to begin with the Fast Track or the Raw Food Revolution Diet? Read through both programs carefully, examine your life honestly, and decide which would be the best fit for you now or in the near future. While the Fast Track is an excellent initiation for anyone, it's especially well-advised if any of the following applies to you:

- You have huge diet changes to make. You eat a diet rich in processed foods, meat, and high-fat dairy products.
- You have a type A personality. You have a sense of time urgency, constant apprehension about impending disasters, and are generally impatient and easily angered.

■ You are prone to addictions or addictive behaviors.

Even if you do not fit into any of the above categories, you may want to choose the Fast Track. Almost everyone will enjoy dramatic health benefits by following the Fast Track, so if you can manage it, we urge you to go for it.

Preparing for the Journey

Regardless of whether you decide to begin on the Fast Track or the Raw Food Revolution Diet, there are several things you will need to do to prepare for your journey.

■ **Get a physical checkup.** Find out about your blood cholesterol, triglyceride, and blood sugar levels. Check your blood pressure and body weight. If you are on prescription medications, make sure that your health care provider knows about your diet plan. You will need to be closely monitored; when people embark on a raw food diet, medications commonly need to be adjusted or stopped completely. This must be done with the approval and assistance of your health care provider. Raw food diets commonly result in weight loss and normalization of blood pressure, blood cholesterol, and blood sugar levels. People who are on medications for high blood pressure, high cholesterol, or type 2 diabetes may notice rapid changes in their condition and their requirements for these medications. Those on insulin or oral hypoglycemic agents need to monitor their blood sugars closely, as blood sugars may drop too low. In this event, your health care provider may choose to prepare a new medication schedule for you. In any case, regular blood sugar monitoring is essential.

■ **Keep a three-day diet and lifestyle record.** Write down everything you eat and drink and try to include at least one weekend day. The following pieces of information need to be included in the record:

- type and amount of food consumed
- time of day you ate the food
- place the food was eaten
- preparation method used
- reason for selecting the food
- degree of physical hunger felt (0 being not hungry; 5 being famished)
- how you felt before eating the food
- how you felt after eating the food

Also keep a record of all addictive substances that you take in (alcohol, cigarettes, or recreational drugs). Note your sleeping patterns: the amount of time you sleep each day, when you sleep, and where you sleep. Note your physical activity patterns and record any fitness activities. Also take note of anything special you did for yourself—enjoyable social activities, massages, meditation, pedicures, prayer time, or yoga classes. Keeping a written record heightens your awareness and, in the process, increases your motivation for making positive changes.

■ **Deliver yourself from temptation.** Get rid of the foods and other items that tempt you. You don't need that kind of pressure. Bring the unwanted items to a food bank or a homeless shelter, or give them to someone you know will be buying them anyway. If others in your household are in opposition to your giving the goodies away, explain to them why you are doing this and why you would be grateful for their support. Perhaps they might be willing eat these foods outside of the home.

■ **Restock your pantry.** Go shopping for the items you will need to prepare all of the delicious recipes you select. Review pages 71–75 and consider investing in some good food-preparation equipment.

■ **Acquire the necessary supplies.** Ideally, you'll need a blender and food processor, and perhaps a juicer; a dehydrator is optional. See pages 78–87 for more information about equipment that is useful in raw food preparation.

■ **Experiment before beginning.** Get acquainted with sprouting (see page 90 for guidelines). If you have access to a juicer, start juicing greens. Play around with the recipes. Get comfortable with preparing raw food.

■ **Build a support system.** Discuss your upcoming journey with family and friends and ask for their support. Get acquainted with local support groups. Attend raw food events, raw food potlucks, or other raw food activities offered in your community.

■ **Pick a date to begin.** If you are following the Fast Track, you'll want to select three weeks that are free of travel and holiday celebrations. You'll also need to ensure that time is allotted for food preparation, self-care, and stress management. The Raw Food Revolution Diet is long term, so you only need to decide when you are ready to start.

THE FAST TRACK

The Fast Track is an aggressive and extremely effective program. It provides significant results in a short period of time. Depending on your state of mind, it can be perceived as a boot camp or as a soothing retreat. You'll take in nothing that is physically damaging in any way. Dietary components that harm the human body are basically eliminated in this phase of the plan. You don't have to weigh or measure your food and you don't have to count calories. The Fast Track lasts only three weeks, so there's no long-term commitment. The three-week time frame was selected because researchers have discovered that it takes about three weeks to rewire your taste buds and break bad habits. Unless you have access to a raw food restaurant or a restaurant with plenty of salad items or a salad bar, it's best to avoid eating out during this three-week period.

Eating on the Fast Track

The Fast Track phase is 100% raw. The good news is that you don't have to cook for three weeks! You still will have some food preparation to do, although it can be minimal if you choose.

Five of the menus on pages 92–100 are designed to meet the Fast Track guidelines. The only menu that is not 100% raw is Menu 3. In this menu, 1 cup (250 mL) of cooked legumes is included, boosting protein without adding fat. (All six menus are entirely suitable for the Raw Food Revolution Diet program as well.)

FOODS ALLOWED (NO RESTRICTIONS)

- raw vegetables
- raw fruits
- sprouted grains
- sprouted legumes

FOODS ALLOWED IN LIMITED QUANTITIES AS LISTED

- raw, unsalted nuts: ¼ cup/160 mL (about 1 ounce/28 g) per day
- raw, unsalted seeds: ½ cup/120 mL (about 2 ounces/56 g) per day
- flaxseed oil or suitable alternative (see page 48): 2 teaspoons (10 mL) per day
- vegetable juices (2 cups/500 mL) per day
- smoothies (3 cups/750 mL) per day

BEVERAGES ALLOWED (NO RESTRICTIONS)

- water (filtered or purified)
- herbal teas (caffeine free)

Additional Guidelines

Include a multivitamin/mineral supplement as well as calcium and vitamin D supplements each day (see chapter 3 for more information).

Avocados and olives are avoided during this part of the program, as they are high in calories and don't include enough of the other essential nutrients to warrant their inclusion during this intensive weight-loss phase.

Nuts and seeds are included (in limited quantity), although they are high in fat and calories. These foods are rich in nutrients, including protein, vitamin E, and trace minerals. It would be a challenge to meet the recommended intakes for these nutrients without nuts and seeds.

Concentrated fats and oils are generally avoided. The only exception is up to 2 teaspoons (10 mL) of a high-quality omega-3-rich oil, such as flaxseed, hempseed, or other oil with at least as much omega-3 fatty acids as omega-6. This can help to ensure that your requirements for omega-3 fatty acids are met and a healthful balance of essential fatty acids is maintained. Although oil rich in omega-3 fatty acids is permitted, it's not necessary, as essential omega-3 fatty acids can be supplied by nuts and seeds, such as walnuts, flaxseeds, and hempseeds.

Concentrated sweets and sweeteners are also generally avoided during this phase.

The Fast Track Lifestyle

Sleep

Adequate rest is important to optimal health throughout life and is critical to the success of the Fast Track. We recommend a full eight hours a night, if possible. If you need more, plan for it. If eight hours is too much for you, aim for at least seven hours. Listen to your body. Don't rob yourself of rest, as it will compromise your performance both physically and mentally. Research has demonstrated that sleep deprivation results in adverse changes to the appetite-control hormones and contributes to weight gain.

Like any other aspect of health, sleep requires some preparation. Activities that calm and soothe, such as a warm bath and an enjoyable book, are good choices. Many people find that eating their last meal several hours before bedtime works best, so as not to interfere with sleep. Some need a light bedtime snack to sustain their blood sugar levels. Get into the habit of a regular bedtime hour and stick to it as much as possible. It's important that our place of rest be free of light and noise. If you live close to a fire station and in a highly lighted area, consider investing in good blinds, earplugs, and an eye mask. Do whatever you can to make your place of rest one that is peaceful and inviting.

Exercise

The Fast Track is not the time to leap into an extreme fitness program. Remember, you're working on rewiring your system. However, do include a moderate, regular exercise regimen. As you move on to the Raw Food Revolution Diet, you can increase the intensity and duration of your fitness routine. For now, stick to yoga, brisk walking, hiking, jogging, fitness classes, or any other activities you normally do. This is a great time to add a good stretching routine to your regimen.

Sunshine

Many people view the sun as something to be avoided due to its link to skin damage and skin cancer. Of course, it is important to be conscious of this connection and moderate your exposure. However, it's also important to recognize the healing power of the sun and ensure that you get a regular, reasonable dose. The sun's healing rays may help to prevent depression, osteoporosis, certain cancers (breast, prostate, and non-Hodgkin's lymphoma), and some immune and/or inflammatory disorders. How much sunshine is sufficient will vary depending on what part of the world you live in, the color of your skin, and your general state of health (see pages 50–51 for more information on sunshine and vitamin D requirements).

Stress Management

While you are on the Fast Track, pamper yourself without using food. Treat yourself to regular massages. Read a good book. Enjoy your favorite calming music. Have a bubble bath. Take time to pray or meditate. Go for a long walk in your favorite place. Avoid the hustle and bustle of everyday life as much as is possible. Postpone stressful shopping trips unless they are absolutely necessary. Socialize only with people with whom you feel comfortable. Be calm. Be kind. Get to know yourself all over again.

THE RAW FOOD REVOLUTION DIET

If you've just completed three weeks of the Fast Track and are now beginning the Raw Food Revolution Diet, make your transition gradually. Add small amounts of the foods that were not permitted on the Fast Track. If you're just embarking on your journey with the Raw Food Revolution Diet, welcome! We hope you enjoy the adventure.

Eating on the Raw Food Revolution Diet

When you first start out on the Raw Food Revolution Diet, just consume smaller portions of cooked and processed foods, then systematically reduce the number of servings per day of those foods and replace them with fresh, organic plant foods. For example, try replacing french fries with baked potatoes—or better yet, try lightly steamed yams. Whenever you're in the mood for something that's processed or cooked, think about what else might satisfy you. If you crave sugar or bread, reach for some fruit. Rather than cooking vegetables until tender, try pouring boiling water over them and letting them sit for two to three minutes. For instance, broccoli treated this way will turn brilliant green and be warm and satisfying. Instead of using butter, sour cream, or mayonnaise on vegetables, try a little organic flaxseed oil, garlic-infused extra-virgin olive oil, or mashed avocado with some dulse or high-quality, solar-dried sea salt for flavoring.

> When you're going out to dinner, eat a giant green salad before leaving home so you won't be starving. That will keep you in control of your food choices.

What Percentage of Raw Food Is Good to Start With?

You may decide to eat all raw food most days, then eat mostly salad when going out to eat. When you do eat cooked food, try steamed, braised, or grilled organic vegetables topped with unheated oils, or choose other vegan foods such as beans or baked potatoes. As long as you include a salad, you will still be ahead of the pack. When eating out, take your own salad dressing and a few seeds or other toppings to make your salad more interesting. If you choose not to use your stove, it will be easier to eat raw food at home and only eat cooked food when dining out.

You may find it easy to go for weeks eating all raw food and then want to be more flexible when traveling. You may need the "entertainment" value of a dinner out every so often, and it may be important for you to allow yourself that freedom. One approach when eating away from home is to eat fruit as much you like, then eat lightly cooked vegetables, beans, or potatoes, with a double order of salad. If you make the choice to eat cooked food only when dining out and prepare only raw food at home, it will be much easier in the long run to successfully stay on the Raw Food Revolution Diet.

If you experience food cravings or extreme health issues, you may want to try eating 100% raw food for an extended period of time, because an entirely raw diet will help you break your habits and take control of what you eat.

Let's begin with 12 simple raw rules that will help you to build a diet that leads to great health and a lifelong healthful body weight.

1. Eat your veggies. Vegetables provide us with a unique and marvelous complement of nutrients. They are very low in fat and, of course, are cholesterol free. Vegetables are important sources of carotenoids (all those relatives of beta-carotene that our bodies can make into vitamin A), the B vitamin folate, vitamin C, and vitamin K. They're also primary sources of magnesium, potassium, a wealth of other minerals, fiber, and a host of phytochemicals.

Vegetables have the highest nutrient density of any foods. This means that they provide the greatest nutritional value per calorie. Of the colorful rainbow of vegetables from which to choose, those that stand a head above the rest are dark leafy greens. They are undoubtedly the most powerful of all foods on the planet.

- Select a minimum of six servings of vegetables per day. (One serving of raw vegetables equals 1 cup/250 mL.)
- In this mix, aim for three or more servings of dark leafy greens.
- Enjoy other raw vegetables as desired.
- If including cooked vegetables, it's best to steam them. (One serving of cooked vegetables equals ½ cup/120 mL.)

2. Eat your fruit. Fruit is nature's candy. The nutrients provided in fruit are similar to what we find in vegetables, although the nutrient density is generally lower. Fruit delivers a tremendous dose of antioxidants, with berries and pomegranates serving as the crown jewels. It comes as no surprise that fruits are low in fat and are cholesterol free (with the exceptions of avocados and olives, which are high in fat but still cholesterol free).

- Select at least three servings of raw fruits per day.
- Dried fruits are permissible, but use them in small amounts, as they are very high in naturally occurring sugars. Limit them to ¼ cup (60 mL) per day.

3. Include legumes in your daily diet. Beans, lentils, and peas are the iron, protein, and zinc powerhouses of the plant kingdom. They are also loaded with fiber, which helps fend off hunger between meals. Lentils, split peas, and fresh peas (in or out of the pod) are great choices, as they're extremely low in fat and high in nutrients. Several legumes can be successfully sprouted, including dried whole peas, lentils, mung beans, and chickpeas. Legumes have been shown to lower blood cholesterol levels and improve control of blood sugar.

- Select one or more servings of legumes per day.

- Several legumes can be successfully sprouted, including chickpeas, green peas, lentils, and mung beans. Sprouted legumes make a great addition to salads.

- Most other dried legumes need to be soaked, drained, and boiled. Fresh beans do not require soaking and need much less cooking time.

4. Get acquainted with whole grains. Common examples of whole grains include barley, brown rice, kamut, millet, oat groats, rye and triticale berries, spelt, wheat, and wild rice. Amaranth, buckwheat, and quinoa, although technically not "grass" grains, are used as grains in a practical sense. Intact whole grains are not as nutrient dense as vegetables and fruits; however, they are excellent sources of unrefined carbohydrates and a number of valuable vitamins and minerals, including many B vitamins, chromium, copper, iron, magnesium, manganese, potassium, selenium, vitamin E, and zinc. They are also great sources of fiber, plant sterols, and numerous phytochemicals, such as phenolic compounds and, in some cases, phytoestrogens.

Unfortunately, most people eat grains that are highly processed. This means that almost everything of value to health has first been removed, and often health-damaging products, such as hydrogenated fats, salt, sugar, colors, flavors, and preservatives, are added. When whole grains are ground into flour, flaked, or puffed, they lose some nutritional value and their affect on blood sugar and satiety becomes less favorable.

- The best way to eat grains is intact—either soaked or soaked and sprouted.

- If you cook grains, it's best to steam, slow cook, or boil them.

- Cut and rolled grains are less desirable than intact whole grains.

- Avoid highly processed grains and grain products, particularly those with unhealthful ingredients added.

5. Go natural with avocados, nuts, olives, and seeds. High-fat plant foods, such as avocados, nuts, and seeds, have received a bad rap over the years. Whereas avocados and olives were excluded from the Fast Track, they do deliver vitamins and minerals and are a welcome part of the Raw Food Revolution Diet. Experts now recognize that nuts contain protective nutrients that are particularly important when chronic diseases, such as heart disease, are a concern. Surprisingly, regular nut eaters are not at increased risk for being overweight or for obesity, and nuts have been very successfully incorporated into weight-loss programs.

These high-fat plant foods contain impressive levels of powerful antioxidants, phytochemicals, trace minerals, and vitamins. They are also among our richest sources of the amino acid arginine, a potent vasodilator (something that causes blood vessels to relax or expand, improving blood flow). The fat in avocados, nuts, olives, and seeds is mainly unsaturated, and when this healthful fat replaces damaging fats in processed foods and animal products, positive health benefits can be expected.

- Eat at least two servings of avocados, raw nuts or seeds, and/or olives per day.
  - 1 serving of avocado = ½ small avocado
  - 1 serving of raw nuts or seeds = 1 ounce (28 g)
  - 1 serving of olives = 1 ounce (28 g; 6–8 large olives)
- The best ways to eat nuts and seeds are soaked or soaked and dehydrated.
- Avoid nuts and seeds that have added fat, salt, or sugar.
- Store nuts in the refrigerator or freezer.

6. **Limit added fats and oils**. Fats and oils provide a lot of calories with very few nutrients. They dilute the nutrient density of the diet, making it difficult to meet recommended intakes for a variety of nutrients—and in a weight-loss diet, there is very little room for calories without nutrition. Getting healthful fats in the diet is important, and it's best to get those fats from the whole foods listed above whenever possible.

- Limit use of all added fats and oils to not more than 1 tablespoon (15 mL) per day. Less is better.
- If you use concentrated fats and oils, stick to those with omega-3 fatty acids. Good choices are flaxseed and hempseed oils, as well as oils with at least as much omega-3 fatty acids as omega-6.
- If using other fats and oils, select only those that are freshly cold-pressed, such as extra-virgin olive oil.

7. **Stifle sweets**. The story for sweets is not much different from the story for fats and oils. Concentrated sweets and sweeteners provide a lot of calories with very few nutrients. This means sweets and sweeteners need to be avoided or minimized. While there are several reasons to choose natural, organic sweets over highly refined products, being natural does not make sweets good for you. It simply makes them the lesser of two evils.

- Use fresh and dried fruits as your primary sweeteners. These foods provide sweetness packaged with antioxidants, fiber, minerals, phytochemicals, and vitamins.

- If using commercial concentrated sweeteners, select agave syrup, maple syrup, organic brown rice syrup, or organic evaporated cane juice. Keep quantities to a bare minimum.

- If using noncaloric sweeteners, select stevia.

8. **Drink water.** In addition to being calorie free, water offers numerous benefits for health. Over 70% of your bodily functions take place in water. Dehydration, even mild dehydration (as little as a 1–2% loss of your body weight), can leave you exhausted. Water is essential for flushing toxins out of vital organs, carrying nutrients to cells, and maintaining a healthy metabolism. One recent report, using data from the Adventist Health Study, found that people who consume five or more cups of water per day had remarkably reduced risk for fatal heart attacks or stroke (almost half that of those drinking only one to two glasses per day).

There is a great deal of controversy about what type of water is best. Some people swear by distilled water, while others prefer a filtering system or oxygenated water. There are pros and cons with each choice, and it often depends of the qualities of your region's water supply. Our preference is a good filter that eliminates arsenic, chlorine, fecal coliform bacteria, herbicides, lead, nitrates, parasites, pesticides, other microorganisms, and sulfates, without eliminating minerals, such as calcium and magnesium.

Beware of calorie-containing beverages. Fluids don't fill the stomach the way solid food does, so it's easy to underestimate their contribution to your caloric intakes and your weight battles. If you drink four to five calorie-rich beverages a day, you could take in an extra 500–1,000 calories.

Some people justify the consumption of caffeine-containing beverages by saying that caffeine is an appetite suppressant and it increases the body's ability to burn calories. While there is some evidence to suggest this is true, the effects have been found to be insignificant. Of course, as soon as you start adding sugar and cream to the beverage, even the tiniest advantages would be lost. It's important to remember that caffeine is a stimulant and can increase your heart rate and blood pressure, disrupt your sleep, and cause nervousness and irritability.

The Beverage Effect

- beer: 12 ounces (370 mL) = 110–170 calories
- distilled spirits: 1½ ounces (45 mL) = 110 calories
- fruit juice or soymilk: 8 ounces (250 mL) = 150 calories
- lemonade, fruit punch, or soda pop: 12 ounces (370 mL) = 120–150 calories
- liqueurs: 1½ ounces (45 mL) = 150–190 calories
- mocha cappuccino with whipped cream: 12 ounces (370 mL) = 400 calories, 22 grams of fat (such beverages are essentially liquid desserts)
- milkshake and nonalcoholic eggnog: 8 ounces (250 mL) = 350 calories
- wine: 4 ounces (120 mL) = 80 calories

While some beverages add nutritional value to the diet, you are generally better off eating whole foods, as they provide more fiber and greater satiety. The exceptions are green juices and whole food smoothies. Green juices provide a tremendous boost of highly available antioxidants and nutrients for minimal calories. Smoothies make a healthful meal replacement. To boost the nutritional value of smoothies, add a large handful of greens, such as kale or romaine lettuce. Don't be daunted by the green color—they taste fabulous.

Make clean water your beverage of choice. Individual needs will vary depending on your climate, the liquids you consume from other sources, the moisture in the solid foods you consume, and your level of physical activity.

- For variety and flavor, drink herbal teas or water with a squeeze of fresh lemon or lime juice.
- For added nutrition with minimal calories, include vegetable and/or wheatgrass juices.
- If you do consume nutritious, higher-calorie beverages, such as fruit juices, fruit smoothies, soymilk, and rice or other grain milks, think of them as you would any other food rather than as a beverage to wash food down (and choose nondairy beverages that are fortified with calcium and vitamin D). Fruit smoothies with carefully selected ingredients can make excellent meal replacements. If you use smoothies in this way, limit them to one a day.

9. **Listen to your body**. Learn to respond to natural hunger signals, and avoid the temptation to eat when you are not hungry or deprive yourself when you are famished. Learn to recognize the difference between physical hunger and environmental or emotional hunger. Develop an action plan for dealing with nonphysical hunger. Your food choices should be a reflection of the powerful connection between those choices and your well-being, rather than a function of convenience or habit.

- Plan for regular mealtimes but be flexible. If you're not hungry at your regular mealtime, postpone your meal. If that's not practical, wait until your next meal to eat or eat very lightly.
- Stop eating when you are comfortable but not full. Don't be afraid to leave food on your plate. You don't have to throw it away; you can save it for later.
- Respond appropriately to nonphysical hunger. If hunger is triggered by your surrounding environment, look at changing the environment. If candy, chocolate, or soda pop is too much of a temptation, don't keep them around. If hunger is triggered by emotions, look at ways you could respond differently to emotional challenges. If sadness triggers

eating, talk to someone or write in your journal. If stress triggers your hunger, go for a long walk, take a yoga class, or have a long bubble bath. If anger triggers your hunger, stomp around the block, write a letter to the editor, or take it out on a punching bag.

10. **Eat mindfully**. Mindful eating is about awareness of food and the consequences of our food choices—for ourselves, and beyond ourselves. It's about being fully conscious of how food affects our health, our nature, and our spirit. It's about recognizing the profound connection between every living thing on earth. Eating mindfully means selecting and preparing food in a way that is respectful of its source. It means appreciating every living being involved in getting the food to our table. It means consuming food with a grateful heart.

- Make mealtime special—set the table, light a candle, and play some quiet music.

- Encourage the participation of everyone in your home, and keep the atmosphere cheerful.

- Make food preparation a priority and allow sufficient time for it. All too often, food preparation is rushed and burdensome. You get out of your food what you put into it. When you set aside the necessary time to prepare your food in a peaceful environment filled with love and gratitude, you infuse your food with peace and love.

- Eat slowly. Chew your food well. This will enable you to better appreciate your food. As a bonus, it can help reduce the amount you eat and aid your digestion.

- Learn about the origins of your food. Buy from local farmers and local producers. Avoid eating foods that are products of exploited workers, ecological destruction, or animal suffering.

11. **Build healthful habits**. Examine your habits and replace those that undermine your goals with better choices. Write down your challenges and your aspirations. Take one small step at a time. If you are hooked on 2% milk, switch to 1% for a few weeks, then to skim milk. Next, try replacing dairy milk with fortified soymilk or other nondairy milk, and finally with homemade Almond Milk (page 106). If you end up "backsliding," don't consume yourself with guilt. Instead, work on ways to make your new, healthful habits even more enjoyable.

- Eat regular, moderately sized meals. Skipping meals can compromise your performance and leave you so hungry that you overeat at the next meal. People who eat breakfast burn more calories during the day and perform better than those who don't.

- Watch your portion sizes when eating high-fat foods. One of the fun things about going raw is you can eat a large volume of food and still lose weight. However, concentrated oils are 100 calories per tablespoon (15 mL), whether they are raw or not. Avocados, nuts, olives, and seeds are also packed with calories. That doesn't make them bad foods, but it does make them likely culprits in sabotaging weight-loss efforts when they are overconsumed. Be cognizant when eating these foods, and keep their portion sizes small.

- Be seated when you eat. Always put your food in a bowl or on a plate and, preferably, eat at the table.

- Avoid eating while you are preparing meals. You may need to sip on a cup of herbal tea (such as mint tea sweetened with stevia) if this is a major challenge for you.

- Keep your hands busy while watching TV to avoid snacking. When people eat while watching TV, they tend to be less conscious of how much they consume. You may wish to do a craft, catch up on the ironing, or do some stretching exercises to keep yourself otherwise occupied.

- Practice good oral hygiene. Experts agree that this can add 10 or more years to your life. Your mouth is considered an excellent indicator of overall health. Take good care of it.

12. Take a multivitamin/mineral supplement plus calcium with vitamin D. When you are limiting your food intake, nutrient shortfalls can result. In addition, whole foods diets are often low in vitamin B_{12}, iodine, and vitamin D. A multivitamin/mineral supplement can help to ensure that your vitamin and mineral intakes are above the recommended dietary allowances. While it is possible to meet your calcium needs by eating plenty of greens, nuts, and seeds, it's easy to slip below recommended intakes (see pages 55–57 for more information).

Raw Tips

I don't have a lot of time for food preparation and chewing all those vegetables. Any suggestions?

The answer to both questions is the same—make blended soups and smoothies. It takes only a few minutes to prepare them, and you'll have no messy kitchen to clean! Chewing is important even if you are drinking your dinner, because digestion begins in the mouth. So, even juice, a creamy soup, and smoothies need to be chewed (or sloshed around in your mouth for a few seconds) before swallowing.

Are there any side effects from the Raw Food Revolution Diet?

The physical effects of making a transition to a raw diet vary considerably for each individual, depending on his or her state of health, state of mind, and overall well-being. While some people notice unpleasant side effects initially, others feel better than they have in years. If you jump into a high-raw diet overnight, the side effects are generally more pronounced. For this reason, a gentle transition may be preferable. That is why experimenting with raw food prior to beginning the program can be helpful. After a lifetime of eating foods that are highly processed and high in fat, pesticides, sugar, and caffeine, you may find that a diet rich in fruit, greens, and minimally processed foods causes significant physical changes in your body. Some individuals report experiencing headaches, nausea, rashes, and changes in their gastrointestinal system. This brief discomfort is often attributed to unwanted substances being removed from the body. This process is referred to as detoxification, particularly within the realm of alternative medicine. If you are concerned about your symptoms, you may wish to consult with an alternative medical practitioner, such as a naturopathic physician.

How can I go raw if I live in a cold climate?

Raw food doesn't have to mean cold food. Here are a few hints that will make it easier to eat raw food in winter.

- Enjoy a warming breakfast of Buckwheat Muesli (page 111), Crunchy Buckwheat Granola (page 114), Cinnamon Oatmeal (page 113) with warm Almond Milk (page 106) and bananas, or Sprouted Grain Bread (page 122).

- For breakfast or an afternoon snack, have homemade Almond Butter (page 138) with apples or bananas. If you're brave, sprinkle a generous dose of cayenne on top for an extra kick.

- Use hot water instead of cold water in your smoothies and blended soups.

- Wash your refrigerated produce in warm water or put it in a warm water bath for a few minutes before using it.

- Have a cup of warm miso soup or warm ginger tea before eating your cooler raw meal. This will also reduce your appetite without adding calories.

- Pour nearly boiling water over your refrigerated broccoli or cauliflower and let it rest for a few minutes to warm it up before using it in salads, Crudités (page 174), or other dishes that will be consumed immediately.

- Add some baked or steamed root vegetables or cooked sprouted lentils to your soups and salads.
- Make a warm soup of finely julienned vegetables and hot water. Add Dried Shiitake Mushroom Powder (see page 164), tamari, and grated fresh ginger to boost the flavor.
- Use a dehydrator to warm dishes like raw stuffed mushrooms and marinated kale. Be sure to use a covered glass dish so the item doesn't dry out. Other foods, such as marinated vegetables, can be put in a jar and then immersed in hot water to warm them up quickly before serving.
- Drink a cup of warm ginger tea sweetened with a little agave syrup or stevia before bedtime. It will help you warm those cold sheets.

The Raw Food Revolution Diet Lifestyle

The only lifestyle aspects that change on the Raw Food Revolution Diet from the Fast Track are the exercise and stress management components. The recommendations regarding sleep and sunshine remain the same (see pages 20 and 21).

Stress Management

If you began with the Fast Track, the emphasis on stress management was very high. You were in pampering mode, and you were attempting to reduce stress in your life as much as possible. While it's great to be able focus so keenly on stress reduction or personal pampering, it's unrealistic to expect this to continue indefinitely. Most of us face stressful situations on a daily basis, and while stress reduction can be achieved at some level, it is more important to focus on handling stress, as it's not possible, nor even desirable, to eliminate it completely.

Stress can have very positive consequences for personal growth. Managing stress is about our response to stressful situations. It's our response that most profoundly influences our long-term well-being. Think about how you can improve your responses to stress. Think about incorporating relaxation into your life on a regular basis. There are numerous relaxation techniques to explore, from yoga and meditation to music therapy and massage.

Exercise

Physical activity is essential to optimal health. Unfortunately, it often gets put on the back burner unless it becomes a real priority in your life.

avoid your enemies, know your allies

In the healthy-diet game, there are enemies and there are allies. Get to know them. Never underestimate your enemies; take advantage of your allies.

TOP 10 DIET ENEMIES

1. calorie-laden beverages: alcoholic drinks, fancy coffees, milkshakes
2. deep-fried foods: french fries, fried chicken, fried fish, onion rings
3. fatty meats: hamburger, pork chops, spare ribs
4. high-fat dairy products: cheese, cream, cream cheese, ice cream, sour cream, whipping cream, whole milk
5. high-salt convenience foods: canned and pre-packaged soups and stews, macaroni and cheese in a box, ramen noodles
6. processed and canned meats: bacon, salami, bologna, wieners, canned luncheon meats
7. processed foods containing partially hydrogenated fat or lard: cookies, crackers, margarine, pastries, pies, microwave popcorn
8. refined starch products: white flour, white rice, other refined starches, and products made with refined starches (such as breads, cookies, crackers, pastries, pies)
9. refined sugar products: processed foods made with corn syrup, brown sugar, glucose, high-fructose corn syrup, white sugar, and other sugars
10. salty, fried snack foods: cheese puffs, corn chips, potato chips

TOP 10 DIET ALLIES

1. clean water and herbal teas
2. fresh fruits: apples, berries, citrus fruits, grapes, kiwi, papaya, peaches, pears, pineapple, plums, mangoes, melons
3. green leafy vegetables: broccoli, Brussels sprouts, cabbage, Chinese greens, collards, kale, lettuce, mixed wild greens, spinach
4. herbs: basil, marjoram, oregano, parsley, rosemary, sage, thyme
5. high-starch vegetables: corn, potatoes, sweet potatoes, winter squash, yams
6. intact whole grains: brown rice, buckwheat, kamut, oat groats, quinoa, rye, wild rice
7. legumes of all kinds: beans, lentils, and peas
8. nonstarchy vegetables: asparagus, carrots, cauliflower, celery, cucumbers, eggplant, mushrooms, peppers, tomatoes, turnips, zucchini
9. raw nuts: almonds, Brazil nuts, hazelnuts, walnuts
10. raw seeds: flaxseeds (ground), pumpkin seeds, sesame seeds, sunflower seeds

Exercise must be viewed as a necessary part of daily life, like brushing your teeth or going to the bathroom. Your body needs to be challenged if you are to reach a truly healthful body weight. Exercise offers huge advantages when it comes to weight loss. It increases stamina, energy output, and metabolism.

- **Exercise daily.** Your best choice for weight loss and overall health is moderate aerobic activity (such as brisk walking) combined with moderate resistance training (such as light weight training). Don't forget to stretch!
- **Avoid labor-saving devices when you can.** Take the stairs instead of the elevator, park a couple of blocks from work, and hide the remote control.
- **Be adventurous.** Join a hiking club, take tennis lessons, or sign up for kayaking classes.
- **Don't avoid an activity because of your size.** By being active you are setting a great example for others and living life to its fullest.
- **Aim for 30–60 minutes of exercise each day.** If this amount of time is too much for you to start with, try doing several short 10-minute sessions throughout your day.
- **Include a balance of cardiovascular, flexibility, and strength exercises.** All three types of exercise are vital to optimal fitness. Too often flexibility and strength are ignored, and we pay the price as we age.

GETTING ALL YOU NEED FROM THE RAW FOOD REVOLUTION DIET

Now that you that you're equipped with the strategy for success, you might want to know more details about how we put this diet together. It'll give you peace of mind to know that you can get a fully nutritious diet by eating raw food, and you'll get important pointers for ensuring you get everything you need to maintain your health. We provide this information and more in the next chapter, where we'll show you how to put together the building blocks of raw nutrition.

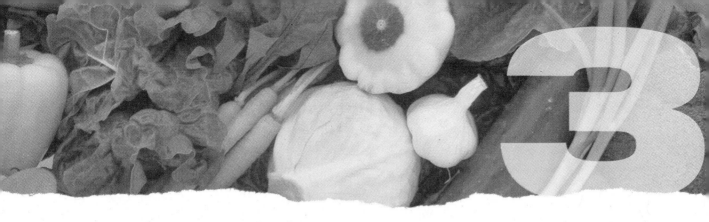

getting the nutrients you need

Our bodies rely on the food we eat to provide an assortment of nutrients; this is no less true while we're losing weight. To achieve and maintain vibrant health, our cells require a steady stream of carbohydrates, essential fats, protein, minerals, and vitamins. Raw diets can be superbly designed to support health and meet our nutrient requirements.

In this chapter you'll learn about how to get the nutrients you need for the Raw Food Revolution Diet path that suits you.

CALORIES

A key attraction of raw and near-raw diets is that they help people shed excess fat while providing antioxidants, fiber, minerals, and vitamins. Vegetables provide more vitamins and other protective nutrients per calorie than other foods. Furthermore, unprocessed raw foods take time to chew, giving the body more time to feel full. By enjoying whole plant foods, fresh from nature, and following the recipes in this book, you can get the nutrition you need with relatively few calories. (For sample menus, see pages 92–100.)

One American research study gives a good look at what happens to people on a raw diet from a nutritionist's perspective. The study reported on 140 adults between the ages of 30 and 79 who had been eating diets that were about 80% raw for 28 months. The women in the study ate an average of 1,460 calories per day, and the men ate approximately 1,830 calories. Their response to the diet was enthusiastically favorable; some of them wanted to lose weight and were successful in doing so. Participants reported

Calories

QUESTION: Which of the following provides more calories: 1 tablespoon (15 mL) of butter or margarine or 10 cups (2.5 L) of romaine lettuce?

ANSWER: The butter or margarine provides 100 calories, whereas a large salad bowl containing 10 cups (2.5 L) of romaine lettuce contains 95 calories. Furthermore, the lettuce gives you 7 g of protein, 5 mg of iron, 185 mg of calcium, and almost twice your recommended daily intake of vitamin C and folate.

Of course, it's likely that you'll prefer more variety than just romaine lettuce! However, this example makes it clear that supersizing your salad offers numerous advantages, particularly when you want to slim down and stay that way. You can enjoy a feeling of abundance with a plate that is heaped with colorful raw veggies and topped with nuts, seeds, and a savory dressing. In fact, you can add a raw dessert and still have consumed fewer calories (and more nutrition) than you'd find in a standard "meat and potatoes" meal or a fast-food combination.

significant improvements in general health and well-being, emotional and mental health, and decreased bodily pain. They attributed these changes to their mainly raw diet. The participants in this study ate five times the American average of 3–4 servings of vegetables and fruits daily. (Serving sizes on food guides are typically equivalent to one apple, banana, or carrot, 1 cup/250 mL of salad, or ½ cup/120 mL of cooked vegetables.) Over the course of a day, study participants ate 11–12 servings of vegetables and 6–7 servings of fruit for a total of 18 servings (1,700 grams) of mainly raw fruits and vegetables. Furthermore, what they ate was far superior in nutritional quality than typical choices on the Standard American Diet, such as fries, ketchup, and iceberg lettuce.

Three-quarters of the calories the study participants ate came from raw foods and one-quarter from cooked grains, vegetables, and legumes. By weight, the diets were 82% raw. Fruits were the biggest contributor of calories. Salads contributed the most nutrition overall. Nuts, seeds, and plant oils were also included in menus and recipes.

The following pointers emerged from this pioneer study of raw food diets:

- Take care not to let caloric intake drop too low.
- Be sure to include nuts and seeds and sprouted or cooked legumes for their valuable contribution of calories, protein, minerals, and vitamins.
- Include a reliable source of vitamin B_{12}. (For more on this vitamin, see page 52.)

Until now, you may not have considered veggies or seeds as significant sources of protein. Prepare for a shift in perspective! In both ground beef and broccoli, 33% of the calories come from protein. (In the beef, all of the remaining calories come from fat, whereas in broccoli, 58% of the calories come from carbohydrate and just 9% from fat). The calories from protein in asparagus, bok choy, lettuce, mushrooms, spinach, and zucchini are found in a similar proportion to broccoli. When you add a seed-based dressing to meals made with these vegetables, you increase the protein content, while the fat content of seeds increases the feeling of satiety.

Calories and Protein in Raw Food

The calories and protein provided by a wide assortment of raw fruits, vegetables, nuts, seeds, legumes, and grains are shown in table 2. This table shows the grams of protein in various foods and also gives the percentage of calories that are derived from protein, carbohydrates, and fat. (The total of these three shaded columns is 100%.) The column to the right shows the percentage by weight of the food that is water. As water contains no calories at all, items with a high-water content are valuable plate fillers when you want to lose weight!

When you are not trying to lose weight, your diet should provide at least 10% of calories from protein. While you're trying to lose weight and your caloric intake is somewhat low, you will have the best success if at least 12–20% of your calories comes from protein. The foods that grow in pods (beans, edamame, lentils, peas, and other legumes) are the most concentrated plant protein sources, with 23–32% of their calories coming from protein. Thus legumes are nature's protein powerhouses; they quickly boost our protein intake. Seeds range from 11 to 17% of calories from protein, with pumpkin seeds at the high end. Nuts contain 8–15% calories from protein, and grains 9–18%. Vegetables vary a great deal, from yams (5% calories from protein) to baby zucchini (40% calories from protein). Fruits provide relatively little protein. As you can see at the bottom of table 2, oils are protein free.

Avocado, coconut, dried fruit, durian, olives, nuts, seeds, and nut or seed butters are concentrated sources of calories. Grains and legumes can boost your energy intake while being relatively high in protein. While the focus of this book is on weight loss and management, note that it's possible to design raw and mainly raw diets that meet the needs of people with high activity levels and big appetites. So if your goal is weight loss or weight management, yet you share mealtimes with people whose dietary goals are entirely different, they still can benefit from the high intakes of protective vitamins, minerals, and phytochemicals in raw foods and follow a diet that meets their requirements.

PROTEIN

 e require protein for the maintenance of muscle, blood cells, bone, and cells throughout the body. Proteins and amino acids (the building blocks of protein) make up the enzymes

calories and protein in raw foods

TABLE 2 · Percentage of calories from protein, fat, and carbohydrate; and percentage of water*

FOOD	CALORIES PER CUP OR UNIT	PROTEIN PER CUP OR UNIT, GRAMS	PERCENTAGE OF CALORIES FROM PROTEIN	PERCENTAGE OF CALORIES FROM CARBO-HYDRATES	PERCENTAGE OF CALORIES FROM FAT	PERCENTAGE OF WATER
FRUITS						
Apple, medium-size, each (138 g)	72	0.4	2	95	3	86
Apples, dried, cup (160 g)	440	4	4	96	0	26
Apricot, each (36 g)	17	0.5	10	83	7	86
Apricots, dried, cup (160 g)	429	6	5	93	2	30
Banana, dried, cup (100 g)	346	4	4	92	4	3
Bananas, medium-size, each (126 g)	110	1	4	93	3	75
Blackberries, cup (144 g)	62	2	12	79	9	88
Blueberries, cup (145 g)	82	1	5	90	5	84
Blueberries, dried, cup (160 g)	560	4	3	97	0	10
Cantaloupe, diced, cup (156 g)	53	1	9	86	5	90
Cherimoya fruit, cup (225 g)	211	3	5	92	3	74
Coconut milk, cup (240 g)	552	6	4	9	87	68
Coconut, dried, cup (116 g)	766	8	4	13	83	3
Currants, European/black, cup (112 g)	71	2	8	87	5	82
Dates, pitted, chopped, cup (178 g)	502	4	3	96	1	21
Durian, chopped, cup (243 g)	357	4	4	66	30	65
Fig, medium-size, 2¼ inch (6 cm), fresh, each (50 g)	37	0.4	4	93	3	79
Figs, dried, cup (199 g)	496	7	5	92	3	30
Grapefruit juice, cup (247 g)	96	1	5	93	2	90
Grapefruit, each (246 g)	103	2	7	90	3	88
Honeydew melon, diced, cup (170 g)	61	0.9	5	92	3	90
Kiwi, medium-size, each (76 g)	46	0.9	7	86	7	83
Mango, dried, cup (121 g)	424	0	0	100	0	14
Mango, each (207 g)	135	1	3	94	3	82
Orange juice, cup (248 g)	112	2	6	90	4	88
Orange, medium-size, each (131 g)	62	1	7	91	2	87
Papaya, cubes, cup (140 g)	55	0.8	6	91	3	89
Peach, dried, each (13 g)	37	0.7	7	93	0	30
Peach, medium-size, each (98 g)	38	0.9	8	87	5	89
Pear halves, dried, cup (180 g)	472	3	3	95	2	27
Pears, medium-size, each (166 g)	100	1	4	88	8	83

FOOD	CALORIES PER CUP OR UNIT	PROTEIN PER CUP OR UNIT, GRAMS	PERCENTAGE OF CALORIES FROM PROTEIN	PERCENTAGE OF CALORIES FROM CARBO-HYDRATES	PERCENTAGE OF CALORIES FROM FAT	PERCENTAGE OF WATER
Pineapple, diced, cup (155 g)	74	0.8	4	94	2	86
Plum, each (66 g)	40	0.5	5	86	9	84
Plums, dried, cup (121 g)	273	3	4	96	0	36
Prunes, dried, cup (170 g)	408	4	4	95	1	31
Raisins, seedless, packed, cup (165 g)	493	5	4	95	1	15
Raspberries, cup (123 g)	64	1	8	82	10	86
Strawberries, whole, cup (144 g)	46	1	8	85	7	91
Watermelon, cup (152 g)	46	0.9	7	89	4	91
VEGETABLES						
Asparagus, each (19 g)	5	0.4	35	62	3	93
Avocado, all varieties, each (201 g)	324	4	5	78	17	74
Basil, fresh, chopped, cup (42 g)	11	1	31	52	17	91
Beans, snap green/yellow, cup (110 g)	34	2	20	77	3	90
Beet juice, cup (236 g)	83	3	12	88	0	88
Beets, sliced, cup (136 g)	58	2	14	83	3	88
Bok choy, shredded, cup (70 g)	9	1	36	53	11	95
Broccoli florets, cup (70 g)	20	2	33	58	9	91
Cabbage, Napa, chopped, cup (85 g)	15	1	29	71	0	92
Cabbage, red, chopped, cup (89 g)	28	1	16	80	4	90
Carrot juice, cup (236 g)	50	1	11	83	6	93
Carrot, 7½ inch (19 cm), each (72 g)	30	0.7	8	87	5	88
Cauliflower florets, cup (100 g)	25	2	26	71	3	92
Celery root, chopped, cup (156 g)	66	2	13	81	6	88
Celery, large stalk, 11–12 inches (28–30 cm), each (64 g)	9	0.4	17	74	9	95
Cilantro, cup (46 g)	11	0.9	27	58	15	92
Corn, yellow/white, cup (154 g)	132	5	13	76	11	76
Cucumber, peeled, each (201 g)	24	1	19	69	12	97
Dandelion greens, chopped, cup (55 g)	24	1	20	68	12	86
Eggplant, cubed, cup (82 g)	20	0.8	14	80	6	92
Garlic cloves, each (3 g)	5	0.2	16	81	3	59
Green Giant Juice (page 119), cup (250 g)	38	3	36	57	7	96
Horseradish, cup (240 g)	144	7	18	78	4	77
Kale, chopped, cup (67 g)	34	2	22	67	11	84
Kelp, Japanese, chopped, cup (80 g)	34	1	14	76	10	82

(continued)

FOOD	CALORIES PER CUP OR UNIT	PROTEIN PER CUP OR UNIT, GRAMS	PERCENTAGE OF CALORIES FROM PROTEIN	PERCENTAGE OF CALORIES FROM CARBO-HYDRATES	PERCENTAGE OF CALORIES FROM FAT	PERCENTAGE OF WATER
Leeks, chopped, cup (89 g)	54	1	9	87	4	83
Lettuce, butterhead/Boston/Bibb, chopped, cup (55 g)	7	0.7	33	55	12	96
Lettuce, leaf, chopped, cup (56 g)	8	0.8	30	62	8	95
Lettuce, romaine, chopped, cup (56 g)	10	0.7	24	63	13	95
Mushrooms, shiitake, dried, cup (145 g)	483	38	31	62	7	12
Olives, ripe, 1 cup (160 g)	206	2	4	6	90	80
Onions, green, each (5 g)	5	0.3	19	77	4	90
Onions, chopped, cup (160 g)	67	1	8	90	2	89
Parsley, cup (60 g)	22	2	27	57	16	88
Parsnips, sliced, cup (133 g)	100	2	6	91	3	80
Pea pods, snow/edible, cup (63 g)	26	2	26	70	4	89
Peas, cup (145 g)	117	8	26	70	4	79
Peppers, hot green chile, cup (150 g)	60	3	17	79	4	88
Peppers, hot red chile, cup (150 g)	64	3	15	65	20	88
Peppers, sweet/bell, red, medium-size, each (119 g)	31	1	13	78	9	92
Radish sprouts, cup (38 g)	16	1	29	28	43	90
Radish, medium-size, each (4.5 g)	4	0	16	79	5	95
Spinach, chopped, cup (30 g)	7	0.9	39	49	12	91
Spirulina, dried, cup (80 g)	345	68	58	24	18	5
Squash, butternut/winter, cubes, cup (240 g)	108	2	8	90	2	86
Sweet potato, cubes, cup (133 g)	101	2	8	91	1	80
Tomatoes, cherry, each (17 g)	3	0.2	17	74	9	95
Tomatoes, each (149 g)	27	1	17	74	9	95
Tomatoes, sun-dried, cup (54 g)	139	8	18	73	9	15
Turnip, cubes, cup (130 g)	36	1	12	85	3	92
Yam, cubes, cup (150 g)	177	0.8	5	94	1	70
Zucchini, baby, each (11 g)	2	0.3	40	47	13	93
NUTS AND SEEDS						
Almond butter, cup (256 g)	1,620	39	9	13	79	1
Almonds, cup (142 g)	850	29	13	13	74	5
Brazil nut, large, each (4 g)	31	0.7	8	6	86	3
Cashew butter, cup (256 g)	1,503	45	11	18	71	3
Cashew nuts, cup (130 g)	736	24	12	18	70	5

FOOD	CALORIES PER CUP OR UNIT	PROTEIN PER CUP OR UNIT, GRAMS	PERCENTAGE OF CALORIES FROM PROTEIN	PERCENTAGE OF CALORIES FROM CARBO-HYDRATES	PERCENTAGE OF CALORIES FROM FAT	PERCENTAGE OF WATER
Chia seeds, dried, cup (160 g)	784	25	12	34	54	5
Flaxseeds, cup (176 g)	792	40	14	23	63	7
Flaxseeds, ground, cup (128 g)	576	27	14	23	63	7
Hazelnuts, dried, cup (135 g)	848	20	9	10	81	5
Pecans, cup (108 g)	768	10	5	7	88	4
Pine nuts, dried, cup (136 g)	915	19	8	7	85	2
Pistachio nuts, cup (128 g)	713	26	14	19	67	4
Poppy seeds, cup (134 g)	716	24	13	17	70	7
Psyllium seeds, cup (156 g)	367	2	2	8	90	0
Sesame tahini, cup (240 g)	1,421	42	11	14	75	3
Sunflower seed butter, cup (256 g)	1,482	50	13	18	69	1
Sunflower seeds, cup (144 g)	821	33	15	12	73	5
Walnuts, English, chopped, cup (120 g)	785	18	9	8	83	4
LEGUMES						
Adzuki beans, dried, cup (197 g)	648	39	24	75	1	13
Lentil sprouts, cup (77 g)	81	7	28	68	4	67
Mung bean sprouts, cup (104 g)	31	3	32	63	4	90
Snow peas, cup (60 g)	25	2	26	70	4	89
GRAINS						
Amaranth, cup (195 g)	729	28	15	70	15	10
Barley, cup (184 g)	631	23	14	80	6	9
Buckwheat sprouts, cup (33 g)	65	2	14	80	6	48
Kamut, cup (188 g)	692	24	14	82	4	9
Millet, cup (200 g)	756	22	12	78	10	9
Oat groats, cup (164 g)	610	21	13	73	14	10
Quinoa, cup (170 g)	636	22	14	72	14	9
Rye, whole, cup (169 g)	566	25	16	78	6	11
Wheat sprouts (108 g)	213	8	15	80	5	48
Wheat, hard red, cup (192 g)	631	30	18	78	4	13
Wild rice, cup (160 g)	571	24	16	81	3	8
OILS						
Oil, flaxseed, cup (218 g)	1,923	0	0	0	100	0
Oil, olive, cup (216 g)	1,909	0	0	0	100	0

*Source: USDA National Nutrient Database (online at www.nal.usda.gov/fnic/foodcomp/search) and ESHA Research "The Food Processor" nutritional analysis program (www.esha.com/foodprosql).

Protein Recommendations

How much protein does your body need? The answer can be expressed in two ways. First, recommended protein intakes can be expressed in grams (g) of protein per kilogram (kg) of body weight. Based on extensive research, the recommended dietary allowance (RDA) for adult protein intake has been set at 0.8 g protein per kg body weight per day. (This figure includes a safety margin to allow for individual differences.)

To calculate your own specific recommended protein intake, divide your weight in pounds (lb) by 2.2 to give your weight in kg. (This is because 1 kg = 2.2 lb.) Then multiply your weight in kg by 0.8 g of protein per kg body weight to find your recommended protein intake. Table 3 shows recommended protein intakes for several body weights, which are given both in pounds and kilograms.

TABLE 3 Recommended protein intake for selected body weights

BODY WEIGHT IN POUNDS	BODY WEIGHT IN KILOGRAMS	RECOMMENDED PROTEIN GRAMS AT 0.8 G PROTEIN/KG
105 lb	48 kg	38 g
120 lb	54 kg	44 g
135 lb	61 kg	49 g
150 lb	68 kg	55 g
165 lb	75 kg	60 g
180 lb	82 kg	65 g
195 lb	89 kg	71 g

our bodies use to carry substances across cell membranes and the hormones that regulate many body functions. While you lose weight, your protein needs remain fairly constant, yet your caloric intake drops. In other words, when you consume fewer calories, more of those calories must come from protein. You can use the formula to the left to calculate the amount of protein your body needs, and you can also estimate this from the values in table 3.

A good way to boost your protein intake while keeping your fat intake low is to include some of the small legumes, such as green peas in or out of the pod, or to add some cooked legumes (beans, peas, and lentils) to a predominantly raw diet. Sprouted mung beans and lentils can boost your protein intake significantly while being very low in fat. We get the proper mix of all essential amino acids we need by eating a variety of plant foods.

To see the amount of protein in several raw food menus, see chapter 5. To get all the protein you need and still lose weight, you'll have to limit oils, sugars, and syrups; these ingredients entirely lack protein. Focus instead on whole foods such as seeds, nuts, avocado, and olives for your fats, and on fresh and dried fruits as sweet treats.

Another way of comparing your protein intakes is in terms of the percentage of calories you eat from protein. It's recommended that a minimum of 10% of your calories come from protein. (Guidelines from the World Health Organization also advise that 55–75% of our calories should come from carbohydrates, and up to 35% from fat.) A glance at table 2 shows that this balance can be achieved using an assortment of raw foods.

When you eat fewer calories, your recommended intake of protein, in grams, remains the same. So the percentage of total calories that you should get from protein will be somewhat higher than 10%; otherwise, you might lose not only weight but muscle mass as well. Each gram of

QUESTION: You can get about 15 grams of protein in foods such as a hamburger patty, a veggie burger, or a hearty bowl of lentil soup. How will you get this much protein on a raw diet?

ANSWER: Many raw recipes and combinations in this book provide 15 grams of protein. Here are examples for your breakfasts, lunches, and suppers:

- 1 serving of Multi-Grain Cereal (page 112)
- 1 serving of Sprouted Multi-Grain Bread (page 123)
- ¾ cup (180 mL) of Broccoli-Tahini Pâté (page 144)
- 1 serving of Green Garden Salad Bar (page 177) with Tahini-Ginger Dressing (page 154)
- 2 cups (500 mL) of Garden Blend Soup (made with sunflower seeds; page 188)
- 2 cups (500 mL) of Green Giant Juice (page 119) plus ⅓ cup (80 mL) of nuts and seeds
- Caesar Salad with Creamy Horseradish Dressing (page 178), plus 2 Pizza Flax Crackers (page 129)
- 1 serving of Garden Pizza (page 202) with a Sprouted Seed Crust (page 132)
- 1 serving of Fresh Pea Soup (page 187), plus a few Figgie Nut'ins (page 212) for dessert

You'll get even more protein from a serving of Buckwheat Muesli (21 grams protein; page 111), a hearty serving of Creamy Kale-Apple Soup (17 grams protein; page 186), or Vietnamese Salad Rolls (16 grams protein; page 205).

protein provides 4 calories; to get 50 grams of protein on a 2,000-calorie-per-day diet, you'll need 10% of your calories to come from protein (50 grams of protein x 4 calories per gram = 200 calories). On a 1,600-calorie-per-day diet, to get 50 grams of protein you'll need 12.5% of your calories to come from protein.

CARBOHYDRATES

C arbohydrates have received plenty of bad press in recent years. However it's important to distinguish between *refined* carbohydrates (such as white flour and sugar, which are linked with a myriad of health problems) and *unrefined* carbohydrates, which are present in whole plant foods.

To get an idea of carbohydrate sources in raw food, see the column "Percentage of calories from carbohydrates" in table 2 (page 38). Carbohydrate is our ideal energy source and is essential fuel for the brain. In fact, we require a minimum of about 130 grams of carbohydrate per day. Vegetables provide carbohydrate with blends of starches and fiber that help to keep our blood sugar levels steady. The natural sugar in fruits gives us a pleasant lift. In both vegetables and fruits, the carbohydrate is packaged with valuable fiber, phytochemicals, minerals, and vitamins.

Fiber

Fiber is a unique category of carbohydrate because it passes through our intestinal tract undigested. All plants contain fiber—it's what gives them their structure. On the other hand, animals get structure from bones; thus animal products, such as meat and dairy products, are fiber free. Fiber is especially valuable when you want to shed a few pounds, because it helps you feel full and satisfied after a meal. Research indicates that we also may absorb fewer calories when our diets are rich in high-fiber plant foods. Fiber helps to protect us against almost every major chronic disease, including certain types of cancers, gastrointestinal diseases, heart disease, hypoglycemia, and type 2 diabetes.

Plant foods provide several different types of fiber, each of which is chemically unique. Scientists often classify fiber into one of two categories, depending on their viscosity and solubility in water: viscous (soluble) fiber and nonviscous (insoluble) fiber.

Viscous fiber includes gums, pectins, and mucilages. These are gel-forming fibers that become sticky when mixed with water. The best sources of viscous fiber are barley, legumes, oats, peas, seeds, and some fruits and vegetables. Viscous fiber helps to control blood sugar levels, improve insulin sensitivity, and reduce blood cholesterol levels. In recipes, these sticky substances thicken and gel sauces and stabilize salad dressings, preventing them from separating.

Nonviscous fiber includes structural fibers such as celluloses, some hemicelluloses, and lignins. When mixed with water, nonviscous fiber absorbs the water but does not dissolve or become gluey. Wheat bran is among the richest sources of nonviscous fiber, but almost all whole plant foods are good sources. Nonviscous fiber helps keep the gastrointestinal system clean and healthy by adding bulk to the stool and ensuring that foods pass quickly and easily through the intestinal tract. It may also afford protection against colorectal and esophageal cancers.

The recommended minimum amount of fiber is 25 grams per day for women and 38 grams per day for men; these amounts have been shown to provide protection against coronary artery disease. Whereas most North American diets are low in fiber, recommended intakes are easily achieved on raw diets.

Your intestine contains about three hundred different types of bacteria (also known as intestinal flora). Some of these microorganisms partner with your immune system and play powerful roles in supporting your health and protecting you from disease; these are known as friendly flora. Others promote disease. When you increase your intake of raw plant food, the balance of bacteria in your intestines changes and the friendly flora are sustained and fed. In contrast, refined sugar supports the growth of other microorganisms that can be far from friendly to your overall health.

Glycemic Index

The glycemic index (GI) is a way of classifying foods according to how they affect your blood sugar. The GI reflects how quickly the carbohydrate in a food enters your bloodstream, how much it raises your blood sugar, and how long your blood sugar remains elevated. Foods with a high GI often trigger a dramatic upward spike in your blood sugar that tends to be followed by a drop in blood sugar. Foods with a low GI tend to supply the carbohydrate that is a fuel for your brain and body in a gradual and gentle manner; these foods cause a small rise. For example, the GI of the sugar glucose is 100. A GI of 70 or more is considered high, a GI of 56–69 is medium, and a GI of 55 or less is low. To find the GI of a food, a person has to consume enough of the food to provide 50 grams of carbohydrates. The blood sugar response over two to three hours is then charted on a graph. The area under the blood sugar curve is used to determine the glycemic index.

Processing, such as grinding whole grains into flour, typically raises GI. Foods rich in fiber have lower GIs. Viscous fibers, such as pectin (in apples and citrus peel), gums, and the fiber in beans and oats, have been shown to significantly reduce glycemic response. Many other factors, such as acidity, density, and ripeness, also affect GI. Lemon juice added to recipes reduces GI; light, fluffy breads have higher GIs than heavy breads; and ripe fruit has a higher GI than unripe fruit.

While glycemic index can be very useful, it doesn't take into account the amount of food eaten. It's possible to eat only a small amount of a high-GI food but have very little blood sugar response. For example, watermelon has a high GI of 72, but it is relatively low in carbohydrates. If you eat only one piece, the impact on your blood sugar is very small. On the other hand, it's possible to eat a large amount of a low-GI food and get a large increase in blood sugar. This is where the concept of glycemic load (GL) comes in. This is a measure of both GI and the amount of carbohydrates consumed. A GL of 20 or more is high, a GL of 11–19 inclusive is medium, and a GL of 10 or less is low. The glycemic load of a serving of watermelon (120 grams) is 4.

Many of the glycemic index testing results have been rather surprising. For example, the glycemic indexes of some potatoes, rice, and bread are higher than that of ordinary white table sugar. Some people may wonder why low-calorie foods, such as celery, have never been tested. The problem is a technical one for the testers, because it would be difficult to get a volunteer to eat 50 grams of carbohydrates from celery—it's just too much celery to think about! Essentially, from a glycemic index standpoint, celery and other very low-calorie vegetables can be considered as free foods.

Another startling finding is that the GI of fructose and high-fructose foods, such as agave syrup, are considerably lower than the GIs of other sugars. One would naturally assume that this makes fructose and high-fructose syrups the preferred sweeteners. However, recent research suggest that these sweeteners may work against us in our weight-loss battle. It's important to look beyond the glycemic index, especially when a food component has been separated from a whole food and concentrated, as with a syrup. Fructose is metabolized very differently than glucose. Unlike glucose, fructose does not stimulate insulin secretion or enhance leptin production. Because insulin and leptin help to suppress appetite, this suggests that excessive fructose intake may contribute to increased energy intake and weight gain. The take-home message is not that fructose is harmful. When fructose is consumed as a natural sugar in a food rich in fiber and antioxidants (such as fruit), it can reduce blood sugar response and have favorable health effects. However, when fructose is concentrated and consumed in large quantities (such as in soda and other processed foods), it may have very negative consequences for health, including weight gain.

The GIs of a few foods are shown in table 4 (opposite). For additional foods, see www.glycemicindex.com.

Research has shown that people in weight-loss programs are less likely to feel hungry when their diets are centered mainly on whole plant foods with low GIs than when they simply consume less fat. In practical terms, consuming plenty of unprocessed, fiber-rich plant foods staves off hunger pangs and helps you to stay with the program.

FAT

Here's the slim version of the fat story. High-fat diets have long been linked with overweight, obesity, cardiovascular disease, many cancers, and diabetes. In recent years it's become apparent that in addition to quantity, fat quality is a key factor. Specifically, it's best to entirely avoid trans fats (found in hydrogenated fats and dairy products) and to limit intake of saturated fats, for which animal products are the primary sources. On the other hand, essential fatty acids are required for good health, and raw plant foods are rich in these essential fats. Raw natural foods such as avocados, nuts, and seeds and are not

TABLE 4 Glycemic index (GI) and glycemic load (GL) of selected foods

FOOD	GLYCEMIC INDEX	GLYCEMIC LOAD (PER SERVING)	SERVING SIZE (GRAMS)	FOOD	GLYCEMIC INDEX	GLYCEMIC LOAD (PER SERVING)	SERVING SIZE (GRAMS)
SWEETENERS				pear	38±2	4	120
agave syrup	9–12	1	10	pineapple	59±8	7	120
fructose	20±5	2	10	plum	39±15	5	120
glucose	100	10	10	raisins	64±11	28	60
honey	55±5	10	25	strawberries	40±7	1	120
sucrose	68±5	10	7	watermelon	72±13	4	120
FRUIT				**NUTS**			
apple	38±2	6	120	cashew nuts	22±5	2	30
apple, dried	29±5	10	60	**VEGETABLES**			
apricots	57	5	120	beets	64	5	80
apricots, dried	31±1	9	60	carrots	47±16	3	80
banana	52±4	12	120	carrot juice, fresh	43±3	9	1 cup (240 g)
banana, slightly underripe	42	11	120	**OTHER FOODS FOR COMPARISON**			
cantaloupe	65±9	6	120	Alpen Muesli	55±10	10	30
cherries	22	3	120	bread, whole wheat	71±2	9	30
dates, dried	103±21	42	60	chickpeas	28	8	150
figs	61	16	60	lentils, cooked	29±1	5	150
grapefruit	25	3	120	potato, baked (russet)	85	26	150
grapes	46±3	8	120	oat porridge	58	13	250
kiwi	53±6	6	120	rice cakes	78±9	17	25
mango	51±5	8	120	rye crispbread	64±2	11	25
oranges	42±3	5	120	yam	37	13	150
papaya	59±1	10	120				
peach	42±14	5	120				

associated with health problems or with being overweight, perhaps because the fat they contain supports health and is accompanied by beneficial nutrients, such as the antioxidants vitamins A and E, selenium, and phytochemicals.

There are two families of essential fatty acids: the omega-6s and omega-3s, both of which are necessary for good health. Changes in our food supply since the industrial revolution have jeopardized both the quantity and balance of these nutrients. Our current dietary pattern provides excessive amounts of omega-6 fatty acids in relation to omega-3 fatty acids.

Omega-6 fatty acids are present in a great many plant foods and therefore are abundant in raw vegan diets. Fewer foods contain the necessary omega-3 fatty acids; examples are butternuts, chia seeds, flaxseeds (ground), flaxseed oil, hempseed, hempseed oil, and walnuts. Flaxseeds must be ground to allow us to absorb the omega-3s they contain; otherwise these smooth, shiny little seeds simply slide through the intestines. Leafy greens such as kale, lettuce, and spinach are excellent sources of omega-3s if you eat enough of them. For example, you can get your day's supply of 2.2 grams of omega-3 fatty acids from 1 teaspoon (5 mL) of flaxseed oil, 1½ tablespoons (22 mL) of ground flaxseeds, ¼ cup (60 mL) of walnuts, or 18 cups (4.5 L) of kale. A big green salad topped with some walnuts or Liquid Gold Dressing (page 151) will easily do the trick!

You can realize powerful health benefits if you consume enough of these essential fatty acids in the right proportions. Hormonelike substances formed from omega-6 fatty acids tend to raise blood pressure, promote inflammation, cause blot clots, and increase cell division; substances formed from omega-3 fatty acids provide a necessary balance that protects against these responses. In addition, omega-3 fatty acids play important roles in the structure and proper function of cell membranes and are essential parts of our nerves, brain, and retinas of the eyes.

For menus that are nutritionally adequate, meet recommended intakes of protein and essential fatty acids, and will give you "staying power" between meals, see chapter 5.

THE RAW GUIDE TO VITAMINS

When it comes to vitamins, your raw diet will give you a clear advantage; and, with your higher vitamin intake, your cells will gain powerful protection against disease. It's helpful to understand which foods are highest in certain vitamins so that you'll know how get a good balance of the full spectrum of these essential nutrients. (This isn't hard to accomplish!) A few, in particular vitamin B_{12}, and in some geographic locations, vitamin D, require special attention (see page 50).

Antioxidant Vitamins

Raw foods and juices contain spectacular amounts of the antioxidant vitamins, a fact that accounts for their many health benefits. When your cells receive a steady supply of antioxidants, they get the defensive ammunition they need to effectively block free radical damage. The antioxidant vitamins are A (or more accurately, the carotenoids that we make into vitamin A), C, and E. These antioxidants are a formidable line of defense and are team players. For example, vitamin C promotes the activity of vitamin E, and vitamin E protects beta-carotene from oxidation. Antioxidants regularly hit the headlines as scientists investigate the roles of antioxidants in reducing our risk for cancer, cardiovascular disease, cataracts, macular degeneration, diseases of the nervous system (such as Alzheimer's and Parkinson's diseases), and premature aging of skin. Getting our antioxidants from raw plant foods is proving to be far more effective and protective than using antioxidant supplements.

Vitamin A and Carotenoids

Our bodies make vitamin A from beta-carotene, a yellow compound that is abundant in deep yellow, orange, red, and green vegetables and fruits. This vitamin keeps the skin, mucous membranes, and corneas of the eyes healthy. It's required for reproduction and the building and regulation of hormones. Beta-carotene is found in carrots, nori seaweed, peppers, pumpkin, squash, sweet potatoes, tomatoes, turnips, and yams. It's also in fruits such as apricots, cantaloupe, mango, nectarine, papaya, persimmon, plantain, and prunes. In fact, the gorgeous-hued green, orange, red, and yellow vegetables and fruits are sources of more than 50 related compounds known as carotenoids. The one that is most familiar to us is beta-carotene. Carotenoids support the immune system, may protect our cells against cancer and cardiovascular disease, and help prevent cataracts. The carotenoid lycopene gives a red or pink tinge to guava, papaya, pink grapefruit, tomatoes, and watermelon; in our bodies, it reduces our risk of coronary artery disease and various cancers (bladder, cervix, lung, prostate, and skin). Lutein, found in dark leafy greens, such collard greens, kale, mustard greens, spinach, and turnip greens, is associated with the health of our eyes and reduced risk of macular degeneration. In broccoli and other greens, the carotenoids deepen the green hue of the chlorophyll. If you drink a lot of carrot juice, your skin may take on a yellow-orange tone that can last for a week or two; however, this temporary condition is harmless. Because of the abundance of these colorful plant foods, people eating a raw diet usually consume a high level of carotenoids. Typically, we take on a healthy glow without turning yellow!

Finnish researchers found that adults on a raw "living food" diet (see page 12) have larger amounts of the antioxidants alpha-carotene, beta-carotene, lutein, and lycopene in their blood than nonvegetarians.

Vitamin C (ascorbic acid)

Vitamin C helps us resist infection, absorb iron, build thyroid hormone, and form collagen, a protein in blood vessel walls, scar tissue, and bone. Great sources of vitamin C are broccoli, cantaloupe, citrus fruits, leafy greens, mangoes, papayas, peppers, strawberries, tomatoes, and vegetables in the cabbage family. Raw diets typically provide three to six times the minimum recommended level; these amounts likely give us added protection. Cooking has been shown to reduce the vitamin C content of foods by one-third to three-quarters. Finnish researchers found that adults on raw diets have excellent blood concentrations of vitamin C.

Vitamin E (alpha-tocopherol)

Vitamin E is third in the antioxidant vitamin trio. It protects vitamin A and polyunsaturated fatty acids from destruction and has roles in the prevention of many diseases. It stabilizes cell membranes and prevents their breakage. This fat-soluble vitamin is present in avocados, leafy greens, nuts, olives, seeds, and unrefined plant oils such as olive oil. Heat from the oil-refining process destroys vitamin E. In a study in Kuopio, Finland, 21 adults on a diet of berries, nuts, raw fruits, sprouted seeds, and vegetables had vitamin E intakes that were triple the minimum recommended levels. They also had significantly more vitamin E in their blood compared to nonvegetarians who were similar in age, gender, and social status. In weight-loss diets where people eat few avocados, nuts, olives, and seeds, it's difficult to meet recommended intakes for this fat-soluble vitamin, so these natural sources of fat play an important role.

Vitamin D

Vitamin D supports bone density by allowing us to absorb, retain, and use calcium. Current research indicates that a lack of vitamin D may be linked with depression, certain types of cancer, and multiple sclerosis. This vitamin can be supplied both by diet (or supplements) and by sunlight. Making your own vitamin D requires daily exposure of about 10–15 minutes of warm sunlight on your forearms, hands, and face (or an equivalent area of skin surface) if your skin is light-colored. If you're dark skinned, you'll need 2–6 times more sun, or you'll need to expose a greater surface area of skin. At latitudes farther from the equator, there's a "vitamin D winter" for three to five months, with little skin production of vitamin D. Adults in the northern United States and Europe, in Canada, in southern Australia, and in New Zealand don't get enough vitamin D from sunlight during winter months, though visiting a tanning booth can support vitamin D production. When you slather on sunscreen with an SPF of 8 or higher, your skin's production of this vitamin is blocked. It's important to balance your need for vitamin D with common sense; so after a bit of sun exposure, add protective sunscreen. On cloudy days, the energy of ultraviolet rays is cut in half. As you age, your vitamin D production diminishes. By 70 years of age, your skin's ability to produce vitamin D is just 30% as effective as that of a young adult and you're likely to need a supplement or fortified beverage in addition to a little sun exposure. It's important for individuals who are confined indoors to include dietary or supplementary sources of vitamin D.

Raw food sources of vitamin D for vegans include shiitake and maitake mushrooms (when they are dried outdoors, such as under the summer sun for six to eight hours). However, amounts may vary too much to make these mushrooms reliable sources of vitamin D. Foods (that are not raw) that are fortified with vitamin D and are commonly used by vegans include soymilk, rice milk, and breakfast cereals (check labels). Note that vitamin D_3 (cholecalciferol) typically comes from animal sources, such as fish, animal hides, or wool, whereas vitamin D_2 (ergocalciferol) is not of animal origin. Many calcium supplements contain vitamin D in the form of cholecalciferol; some provide the vegetarian form. While scientists have considered vitamin D_2 to be less effective than D_3 at raising serum vitamin D, recent research suggests that there may be no difference in potency.

Vitamin K

Vitamin K helps to build the proteins that allow blood to clot in times of injury. It also regulates blood calcium, giving this nutrient a role in bone health. Vitamin K is found in asparagus, broccoli, cabbage, leafy greens, lentils, peas, and pumpkin; thus it's usually abundant in raw diets. This vitamin is also present in nori, hijiki, and other vegetables from the sea. As a second source, friendly bacteria in your large intestine contribute to your vitamin K supply by manufacturing this vitamin. To support this production, avoid taking oral antibiotics, which can destroy these bacteria, and also limit your intake of sugar, which feeds the microorganisms that compete with our friendly bacteria.

The Energetic B Vitamins

The team of B vitamins is responsible for unlocking energy from the foods we eat. Here are a few of the best sources of each of the busy Bs:

BIOTIN: widely distributed in plant foods

CHOLINE: legumes, nuts, seeds, many other plant foods

FOLATE: almonds, asparagus, avocado, beets, cashews, cauliflower, daikon radish, durian, green vegetables, kelp, kiwi, legumes, oranges, orange juice, parsnips, seeds, shiitake mushrooms

NIACIN: avocado, cherimoya, dried fruit, durian, lentils, mung beans, nuts, peas, seeds, shiitake mushrooms, yeasts

PANTOTHENIC ACID: avocado, buckwheat, durian, figs, grapefruit, Jerusalem artichokes, lentils, plums, shiitake mushrooms, sunflower seeds

PYRIDOXINE: bananas, fruits, many other plant foods

RIBOFLAVIN: almonds, asparagus, avocado, bananas, cashew nuts, durian, nutritional yeast, peas, sea vegetables, seeds, shiitake mushrooms, sweet potatoes

THIAMIN: avocado, carrot juice and carrots, cherimoya, corn, dried fruit, durian, legumes, nuts, peas, seeds, shiitake mushrooms, nutritional yeast

Nutritional yeast is a potent provider of numerous B vitamins. Because riboflavin can be destroyed by light, nutritional yeast should be stored in an opaque container or a dark cupboard.

Vitamin B_{12}

Vitamin B_{12} is presented apart from the other B vitamins because getting enough of this essential nutrient on a raw vegan diet takes a little special care.

Vitamin B_{12} is produced by bacteria in the soil in which plant foods grow. Vitamin B_{12} acts together with other B vitamins to help convert carbohydrate, fat, and protein to energy. It also has a few special roles. It's required for the normal development of red blood cells, to maintain protective sheaths around nerves, and to help build genetic material (DNA). It protects against the buildup of a toxic by-product of amino acid metabolism known as homocysteine, which can increase the risk of heart disease. Without sufficient vitamin B_{12}, the blood is less able to deliver oxygen to the body and fatigue sets in; nerve damage and heart disease can also develop. These symptoms easily can be avoided by ensuring that you have a reliable source of this essential nutrient with a known quantity, specifically a fortified food or a supplement.

OPTION 1. Take 1–2 tablespoons (15–30 mL) of Red Star Vegetarian Support Formula nutritional yeast daily in two doses during the day.

The smaller the form the yeast is in, the more concentrated it will be, so follow these guidelines depending on the type of yeast you use. Each of the following provides your day's recommended intake, which is 2.4 mcg of vitamin B_{12}.

- If using the powdered form, take a total of 1 tablespoon (15 mL) daily.
- If using the mini-flakes, take a total of 1½ tablespoons (22 mL) daily.
- If using the large flakes, take a total of 2 tablespoons (30 mL) daily.

Nutritional yeast is a source of vitamin B_{12} only when it's grown on a medium that contains B_{12}. Vegetarian Support Formula nutritional yeast, produced by the Red Star company, is a reliable source of B_{12}. If you buy nutritional yeast in bulk from a food co-op or natural food store, ask to see the package label to ensure that you are buying this brand of nutritional yeast, especially if you are relying on this as your dietary source of vitamin B_{12}. *Note that we are not referring to baker's yeast (the kind used to make bread) or brewer's yeast.* In contrast to these other yeasts, Red Star Vegetarian Support Formula nutritional yeast provides vitamin B_{12} and it tastes good, with a pleasant, cheesy flavor. You'll find nutritional yeast in certain recipes in this book, such as the delicious Liquid Gold Dressing (page 151).

Though not raw, certain vegan foods, such as fortified soymilk or rice milk, are enriched with vitamin B_{12}.

OPTION 2. Take a daily supplement, such as a multivitamin/mineral supplement, that includes at least 10 mcg of vitamin B_{12}.

When you take your day's supply at once, rather than in two or more doses, you absorb a little less; our recommendation of 10 mcg exceeds the recommended dose for this reason. Most multivitamin/mineral supplements provide at least 10 mcg of vitamin B_{12}. If your food intake is limited, as it may be when losing weight, this choice of a daily multivitamin/mineral supplement has the advantage of providing additional trace minerals and vitamin D.

Meeting Vitamin B_{12} Requirements

If you're on a raw or near-raw diet, you must ensure your intake of vitamin B_{12} by regularly consuming a reliable supply of this essential nutrient, specifically a fortified food such as Red Star Vegetarian Support Formula nutritional yeast or a supplement. Choose one of the following:

- daily, 1–2 tablespoons (15–30 mL) of Red Star Vegetarian Support Formula nutritional yeast divided into two doses
- daily, a supplement that includes at least 10 mcg of vitamin B_{12}
- once a week, a sublingual supplement that provides 2,000 mcg of vitamin B_{12}

vitamin B$_{12}$ imposters

None of the following should be relied on as a source for vitamin B$_{12}$: algae, bits of dirt on produce, fermented foods, intestinal production, mushrooms, probiotics, raw plant foods, seaweeds, spirulina, or sprouts. We obtain little or no vitamin B$_{12}$ from these, or else we receive imposter forms of B$_{12}$ (analogs), which are worse than useless. These analog molecules are not usable to meet human requirements for the vitamin and may even interfere with the action of true vitamin B$_{12}$. These possible sources are unreliable, and the stakes—your health—are far too high.

Ensuring a reliable source of vitamin B$_{12}$ is easily achieved, so it's simple to avoid potential problems. Overall, eating a raw or mostly raw diet will ensure you of a plentiful amount of vitamins, but vitamin B$_{12}$ must be supplemented.

OPTION 3. Take a weekly sublingual (taken under the tongue) supplement that provides 2,000 mcg of vitamin B$_{12}$.

Because a relatively small percentage of a large dose of vitamin B$_{12}$ is absorbed, most of a large dose will not be retained. If a large dose is consumed weekly, the amount should be 2,000 mcg per week. Typically this is a vegan supplement, preferably allowed to dissolve under the tongue rather than swallowed.

Whatever your choice, your actual source of vitamin B$_{12}$ can be traced back to bacteria. (Nonvegetarians also need reliable sources of vitamin B$_{12}$; animal products contain vitamin B$_{12}$ due to bacterial contamination.) Inaccurate information abounds, suggesting that people on raw, near-raw, and vegetarian diets can ensure their intake of vitamin B$_{12}$ without supplements or the use of B$_{12}$-fortified foods, which is not true.

THE RAW GUIDE TO MINERALS

Minerals are key players in many essential body processes, and raw diets provide rich sources of these nutrients. In addition, soaking, sprouting, and fermenting certain foods, such as nuts and seeds, can make it significantly easier for your body to absorb minerals from them. These processes help release minerals that are bound to compounds known as phytates, increasing the proportion of calcium, iron, and zinc that we can absorb.

The fat present in avocados, nuts, olives, and seeds may help with the absorption of certain minerals, and raw food diets can be high in the healthful fats these foods contain. In contrast, a very low-fat diet may hinder the absorption of minerals.

Eating organic foods can supply increased amounts of certain minerals. Though research on this topic is limited, studies have shown that organic crops provide significantly more iron, magnesium, phosphorus, and vitamin C than crops grown using pesticides and herbicides.

Raw food diets can be a wise choice for the budget conscious, delivering more mineral bang for the buck than other ways of eating. French nutritional scientists recently reported that vegetables and fruits deliver extremely good value in terms of the nutrients (such as calcium, iron, and magnesium) delivered per Euro (or dollar) spent. Certainly this would be true in other markets around the world.

Whatever your diet, getting all the minerals you require takes a little planning, but it's well worth the effort. The menus in chapter 5 will give you ideas for how to do this, as they have been designed to meet nutrient intakes.

Minerals constitute about 4% of your body weight. They perform a myriad of functions: as parts of hormones (such as iodine in thyroxine), as central elements in active proteins (for example, iron in the hemoglobin of red blood cells), as transmitters of nerve impulses (calcium, chloride, potassium, and sodium), as essential partners for enzyme activity (magnesium and manganese), and as structural components in bones and teeth (calcium, magnesium, manganese, and phosphorus). In the next few pages, we'll feature several key minerals that require special attention—calcium, iodine, and iron—and give you tips for getting a good supply of minerals in general.

Calcium and Bone Health

Like blood, muscles, and nerves, bones are living tissues. In your bones, calcium and other minerals are constantly being deposited and withdrawn from a matrix, or framework, of protein. These dynamic processes can be compared to the cash flows in a bank. If mineral withdrawals exceed deposits, eventually the reserves are depleted. Though we may think of calcium as *the* bone-building nutrient, in fact, it does not act alone. Calcium is part of a team that also includes the minerals boron, magnesium, manganese, phosphorus, and potassium; the vitamins A, D, and K; and protein. During the first decades of your life, you build bone density, reaching your maximum at about 30 years of age. After that, bone density gradually declines. As an adult, your bone density and bone loss are affected by your intakes of all of these bone-building nutrients, plus your regular participation in weight-bearing exercise. By exercising and centering your diet on these strengthening nutrients, you can maintain the strength and hardness of your bones into old age.

Your best dietary sources of calcium are the following low-oxalate green veggies: bok choy, broccoli, collard greens, dandelion greens, kale, mustard greens, Napa cabbage, turnip greens, and watercress. Note that beet greens, spinach, and Swiss chard aren't included on this list. These latter three greens contain significant amounts of a compound known as oxalate, which can bind calcium (and iron), making these minerals difficult to absorb and unavailable to your body. (In this case, soaking and sprouting don't help release the minerals.) Only about 5–8% of the calcium from these high-oxalate greens is absorbed, compared to 49–61% of the calcium in the low-oxalate greens listed above. (Compare these figures with absorption rates of 31–32% from tofu and from cow's milk.)

Greens are nutritional superstars. They are rich sources of carotenoids, folate, magnesium, vitamin K, and other nutrients. Many are also outstanding sources of calcium.

You can get a recommended intake of 1,000 mg of calcium from your raw diet in a variety of tasty ways. In achieving this, you may have to adjust your meal and snack choices. For example, over the course of a day you could get 1,000 mg of calcium from 3 oranges, 8 figs, ½ cup (about 2 ounces/56 g) of almonds, and 8 cups (2 L) of green salad made from romaine lettuce and some low-oxalate greens (such as finely chopped kale) and served with Tahini-Ginger Dressing (page 154). Table 5 lists another example of how, over the course of a day, you can get 1,000 mg of calcium from an assortment of raw vegetables and fruits. Also see the menus in chapter 5.

TABLE 5 Foods that together supply the recommended daily intake of 1,000 mg of calcium

Food Item	Amount	Calcium (mg)
assorted vegetables (cauliflower, green beans, zucchini)	3 cups/750 mL	80
broccoli florets	1 cup/250 mL	34
Green Giant Juice (page 119)	2 cups/500 mL	207
Sweet Nut'ins (page 212)	4 cookies	174
tossed green salad	3 cups/750 mL	139
watermelon	2 cups/500 mL	20
Zucchini Hummus (page 145)	¾ cup/180 mL	356
Total	—	1,010

To meet recommended intakes, it helps to start your day with Green Giant Juice (page 119), go for the greens at many of your meals, add seeds and tahini dressing to your salads, and snack on figs and almonds. In addition, you can get smaller amounts of calcium from a wide variety of raw plant foods, such as other nuts (Brazil nuts, hazelnuts, walnuts), seeds (flaxseeds, sunflower seeds), basil, carrot juice, celery, prunes, raisins, and oats, so that the mineral contribution from a range of plant foods really starts to add up. When you are past 50 years of age, your recommended calcium intake increases to 1,200 mg. Seniors (in fact, people at any age and on any diet) may find that a simple solution for meeting recommended intakes of calcium can be to "top up" the day's intake with a calcium supplement that includes several hundred milligrams of calcium, plus vitamin D. (For more on supplements, see page 60).

Iodine

Iodine is an essential part of thyroid hormones, such as thyroxine. Thyroid hormones control growth, development, and metabolic rate; they promote bone building and protein synthesis. Thyroid hormones—and the iodine intake upon which they depend—are crucial during pregnancy. Ensuring an adequate iodine intake during pregnancy is extremely important, as this mineral supports normal brain development of the fetus.

Because the amount of iodine in plant foods depends on the amount in the soil in which they grew, the amount of this mineral in foods varies considerably from one region to another. The levels of iodine in soil are related, in part, to the geographic location of oceans and past glaciers. To ensure adequate intakes of this mineral, many countries, such as the United States and the UK, allow table salt to be fortified with it; some countries, such as Canada, require it. About ½ teaspoon (2 mL) of iodized table salt or iodized sea salt delivers the recommended daily intake for an adult (150 mcg). Salt that is not iodized tends to contain little or no iodine, because this mineral is lost in the drying process.

Sea vegetables (seaweeds) provide iodine; however, it can be a challenge to determine how much you are getting. It may be too little; it may be too much. Raw and dried sea vegetables, including kelp tablets and powder, are generally very high in iodine, though the amounts present can vary considerably from one batch to another. For example, quantities are higher in sea vegetables that grow near coral reefs. Iodine in dried kelp can vary eightfold, so that total iodine content varies between 0.1 and 0.8% of the dry weight.

Some raw food enthusiasts use a guideline of ⅒ teaspoon (0.5 mL) of dried kelp per day, or about ¼ teaspoon (1 mL) every two to three days.

It can be a challenge to find a supplier of kelp that has accurate information about iodine content that is available to consumers, although some kelp tablets deliver the amount of iodine stated on the package. It's better to take recommended intakes of iodine in small but frequent amounts (daily, every few days, or weekly), rather than a large dose less frequently.

While sea vegetables provide a range of minerals, phytochemicals, and essential fatty acids, very high intakes of them or other iodine sources can damage the thyroid gland. The Institute of Medicine has set an upper daily limit for adults of 1,100 mcg of iodine.

Iron

It's well-known that iron from plant foods is less efficiently absorbed than the iron present in meat. It's less commonly known that plant-based diets tend to be significantly higher in iron than other diets, so higher overall iron intake can offset somewhat lower absorption. When a meal is rich in both iron and vitamin C, the absorption of iron is increased, compared to a meal with little or no vitamin C. As it turns out, people who center their diets on plant foods have no greater incidence of iron deficiency anemia than do meat eaters.

Raw plant-based diets offer several advantages when it comes to iron absorption. By consuming foods that are high in vitamin C, such as red peppers or citrus fruits, at the same meal or snack with your iron sources, you can double or triple the amount of iron you absorb, because the vitamin C changes iron to a form that is more easily absorbed. The citric acid in fruits such as cantaloupe, citrus fruit, papaya, mangoes, and strawberries further helps this process.

Certain rules about food combining that originated in the 1920s seem to have been based on individual perceptions about digestion. However, these rules have the disadvantage of compromising iron absorption, stating that fruits should be eaten separately from many other foods, including iron-rich foods. If you're considering adopting these rules, here's a better approach: Do some simple challenges on yourself to see if eating various

Excellent Iron Sources*

- almonds, Brazil nuts, or hazelnuts, ⅔ cup (90 g)
- almond or cashew butter, ⅓ cup (80 ml)
- amaranth, dry, 1 Tbsp. (13 g)
- apricots, dried, ⅔ cup (100 g)
- buckwheat, dry, ½ cup (85 g)
- dried figs, raisins, or currants, 1 cup (165-200 g)
- flaxseed, ground, 3 Tbsp. (24 g)
- lentils or mung beans, dry, 2-3 Tbsp. (25 g)
- millet or wild rice, dry, 1 cup (130 g)
- parsley, 1 cup (60 g)
- peas, 2 cups (290 g)
- seeds, ⅓ cup (60 ml)
- sesame tahini, ⅓ cup (80 ml)
- sundried tomatoes, ⅔ cup (36 g)
- spirulina seaweed, dried, 1 Tbsp. (8 g)

*Excellent sources provide at least 3.6 mg iron or 20% of the DRI.

food combinations really does cause digestive problems for you. Listen to your body. It may be that maximizing iron absorption is more critical to your health. If you do notice difficulty digesting certain combinations of foods, avoid those combinations. If you decide to eat fruit separately from your iron-rich meals, be sure to include plenty of vitamin C–rich vegetables, such as broccoli, leafy greens, red peppers, other peppers, tomatoes, and vegetables in the cabbage family, along with iron sources.

Other Minerals

To give you an idea of the mineral wealth of a diverse raw diet, here are plant-based sources of the various other minerals that we need.

CHROMIUM: apples, bananas, barley, grapes, lettuce, onions, oranges, peppers, psyllium seeds, tomatoes, many other plant foods

COPPER: fruit (bananas, prunes, raisins), nuts (Brazil nuts, pecans, other nuts), seeds, sweet potatoes, many other plant foods

MAGNESIUM: bananas, chocolate, cocoa powder, figs, fruits, leafy greens, legumes, nuts, seeds, many vegetables

MANGANESE: berries, pineapple, a wide variety of raw foods

MOLYBDENUM: a wide variety of raw foods

PHOSPHORUS: a wide variety of raw foods

POTASSIUM: bananas, green beans, mushrooms, potatoes, tomatoes, strawberries, plenty of other fruits and vegetables

SELENIUM: asparagus, Brazil nuts, cherimoya, psyllium seeds, shiitake mushrooms, other plant foods

SODIUM (see note below): Bragg Liquid Aminos, celery, tamari, salt

ZINC: cashews, legumes (beans, lentils, peas), seeds, sesame tahini

Note: When it comes to sodium, the intakes of many people are excessive due to their consumption of processed foods high in sodium. In raw diets, sodium is naturally limited to more desirable levels due to an avoidance of salt-laden processed foods.

SUPPLEMENTS AS A SAFETY MEASURE

When you intentionally limit calories in order to lose weight, you need to make nearly every food choice count in order to reach optimum intakes of minerals and other nutrients. At these times, a multivitamin/mineral supplement can help "top up" your mineral intake and will provide vitamin B_{12} (see page 52). Choose a multivitamin/mineral supplement containing chromium and zinc. In addition, take calcium (definitely accompanied by vitamin D), typically as a separate tablet. Multivitamin/mineral supplements generally don't contain enough calcium; otherwise the pill would be too large to swallow. If you prefer not to use conventional multivitamin/mineral supplements, an option may be a whole food green powder supplement with added vitamins and minerals, including vitamin B_{12}, D, and iodine.

Since *most* of what you'll need will come from your raw diet, just one multivitamin/mineral supplement per day, or even every couple of days, plus one calcium tablet will do for most people. Use of a supplement is wise when you're traveling, when you're in circumstances that restrict your food choices, or at times when you're uncertain you're getting everything you need from your diet.

For additional information on general nutrition, essential fatty acids, and vitamin B_{12}, see *Becoming Vegan* and *The New Becoming Vegetarian*, both by Brenda Davis and Vesanto Melina (Book Publishing Company 2000, 2003). For more on the glycemic index, see *Defeating Diabetes* by Brenda Davis and Tom Barnard (Book Publishing Company 2003).

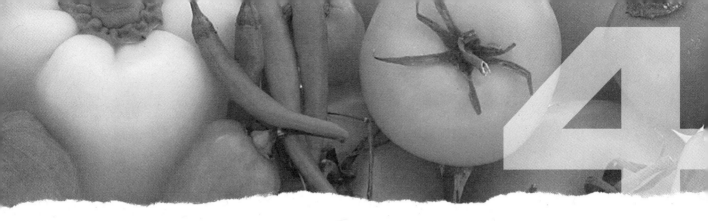

food and equipment basics for the Raw Food Revolution Diet

There are a few common techniques for preparing raw food that will provide more variety to your diet and allow you to take greater advantage of the nutritional content of these foods: juicing, sprouting, and soaking. Although these processes may require a small investment in time and/or equipment, they'll help you enjoy new flavors and get the maximum nutrition from your food. There are a number of excellent books specifically on juicing and on sprouting, but the following information will get you started.

JUICING FOR LIFE!

Juicing is one of the keys to achieving good health and a vibrant life. We could never hope to eat the volume of fruits and vegetables that can fit into one glass when they are juiced and the fiber is removed. That doesn't mean we should remove the fiber from all of our foods, but we can maximize nutrient intake if we include some fresh juices in place of water or other beverages. For some of us, changing to a raw diet is just a matter of including more fruits and vegetables; but for others, a quick switch to eating all that fiber can cause real discomfort. Juicing can make it easier to obtain and absorb the recommended amount of nutrients from our food.

Juicing also allows you to consume vegetables you wouldn't ordinarily eat enough of, like dark greens or wheatgrass, so you can get a wider variety of vegetables in your diet. By combining produce you don't usually eat or can't eat enough of with foods you like a lot, you can increase your nutrient intake and include a full range of foods in your diet.

For recommendations on which juicers to use and how to operate them, see pages 85–86.

Juicing Is as Easy as 1-2-3

1. When you get home from shopping, wash all your fruits and vegetables in a sink full of cold water, dry them, and refrigerate them immediately.

2. Chop or cut your produce into pieces before inserting it into the chute of the juicer.

3. Always drink fresh juice immediately after it has been made, but be sure to chew it first! Making a chewing action when drinking juice gets the digestive juices in the mouth working. Remember that because the cells have been broken down in the juicing process and vitamins are exposed to air, juices not ingested immediately will lose some vitamins due to oxidation.

Wheatgrass and Wheatgrass Juice

Wheatgrass is grown from winter wheat berries, which are the whole kernels, or seeds, of the wheat grain. To the inexperienced eye, wheatgrass looks very similar to common lawn grass. However, considerable differences exist beneath the surface. Many health clinics around the world serve wheatgrass juice to their patients and believe it to be a powerful health elixir.

GROWING YOUR OWN SPROUTS

Sprouts are easy to grow, and nurturing them from seed can be a fun and rewarding experience. Sprouts add texture and flavor to salads and many other raw food dishes. Venture away from familiar alfalfa sprouts and try broccoli, fenugreek, kale, mustard, onion, and radish sprouts.

The process of sprouting grains, legumes, nuts, and seeds greatly increases the bioavailability of the zinc and other minerals they contain. Sprouts are also loaded with phytochemicals and vitamins. They provide a valuable way to get fresh foods during northern winters when little local produce is available, while sailing, or whenever you are far from produce markets.

Basic care of sprouts involves keeping them moist while providing drainage and air circulation. Home sprout growing can be set up with sprout bags, trays, or an automatic sprout grower, but in truth, no special equipment is needed. Wide-neck glass mason jars of any size, plastic screening that can be purchased at any hardware store, and rubber bands for holding the screening in place are all that is required. You can also replace the lids that come with the mason jars with sprouting lids, available at many natural food stores. (These are special lids that have little holes that allow for the necessary drainage and air circulation.)

Regardless of which method you choose, you will more or less follow the same steps. In table 7 (page 90), we summarize what to do for a few of the dried legumes or raw, unhulled seeds that you might like to sprout. Sprouts thrive when they are rinsed often and well drained. In warm weather, they mature more quickly and require frequent rinsing to keep them cool. Hot, direct sunlight can "cook" them; shade is better. To "green" alfalfa sprouts and sunflower greens, a balance of sun and shade works well. In the kitchen, place them on a countertop near a sink to making rinsing and draining convenient.

SOAKING NUTS AND SEEDS

Many people find that soaking nuts and seeds makes them more digestible. Soaking increases the water content of the nuts and reduces the amount of phytates they contain; this is a process that can enhance the absorption of calcium, iron, and zinc. Nuts and seeds should be soaked in water to cover just long enough for them to absorb some of the moisture, but not so long that the minerals are leached into the water. Then rinse off the brackish, often bitter, soaking water. Fifteen minutes to an hour of soaking is usually long enough for seeds, and a few hours is sufficient for nuts, depending on the hardness of the nut. For example, almonds will take longer to soak than walnuts.

If a nut or seed has a brown coating or skin and a slightly bitter flavor, it will benefit from soaking. Good examples are almonds, peanuts, pecans, sesame seeds, and walnuts. Some seeds, such as chia seeds, flaxseeds, and mustard seeds, will develop a mucilaginous quality when soaked, and draining off the soaking water will be difficult to impossible.

Soaking Almonds

Even after almonds are blanched in hot water for a few minutes, they will sprout. To remove the skins from unsoaked almonds, place them in nearly boiling water for up to 5 minutes, or until the skin pops off easily when you pinch an almond between your thumb and forefinger. Once the skins are removed, place the almonds in cold water and allow them to germinate for 8–10 hours. You may store them in the refrigerator immersed in water for up to a week; change the water every other day.

Soaked and Dehydrated Nuts

Many nut pâtés, nut butters, and certain crusts or cookies use nuts that have been soaked and then dehydrated to remove the water. Moist soaked nuts will cause nut butters or pâtés made with them to clump rather than become a creamy spread. To dehydrate soaked nuts, spread them on a dehydrator tray (without the use of a nonstick sheet) and allow them to dry until crunchy, which should take between 8 and 12 hours. Dehydration times vary for many reasons, such as the hardness of the nut or seed (for example, almonds are harder than sunflower seeds and thus take longer to dehydrate), how long they were soaked and therefore how much water they are holding, and the room temperature and humidity.

With a little experience, you will know which nuts and seeds to soak and when not to soak them at all. If you use soaked nuts and seeds on a weekly basis, you may want to keep some soaking in the fridge so they are handy when you need them. Most will stay fresh for several days in the refrigerator after they have been soaked and drained; store them in a sealed glass jar.

FRUIT

Modern science indicates that a nutritious, well-balanced diet should include a variety of ripe, organic fruits. Fruit will not slow you down the way many other foods will, especially fatty foods. That makes them a great choice to eat throughout the day. Most people maintain more energy and better clarity of mind if they eat a light lunch centered mainly on fruits and green vegetables.

Most of us think of fruit as sweet, but cucumbers, eggplant, peppers, squash, tomatoes, and anything containing seeds are also fruits. Examples of savory fruit dishes include avocados or tomatoes filled with Salsa Fresca (page 139) and delicious, savory fruit soups (see pages 186 and 192). Most fruits are a good source of natural sugar for fuel, so sweet fruits prepared in a savory way are an excellent choice for active people.

Ripening and Storing Fruit

Pampering your fruit is pampering yourself—so learning how to care for it is well worth the effort. Choosing and storing fruit with care ensures that you will have ripe, sweet fruit when you want it.

Unripe fruits have not fully developed their sugars and are either tart or less flavorful than mature fruits. If they are consumed while green, they can cause bloating, constipation, and stomachaches. Fruits and other plant foods do not offer optimal nutrition when they are underripe or when they are overripe, so always wait to allow fruit to ripen before eating it and learn how to recognize when each fruit is at its peak of ripeness.

The ambient temperature at which fruit is stored is most often what causes ripening times to vary. Try storing your fruit in different rooms of your house in order to determine which areas have the best temperature for each variety. Warm temperatures cause fruit to ripen more quickly than cooler temperatures. As a general rule, nonsweet fruits, like cucumbers, peppers, and squash, require refrigeration, and sweet fruits do not. Nonsweet fruits, such as cucumbers, peppers, and tomatoes, lose their appealing texture when frozen.

AVOCADOS. Avocados need special care to ensure you'll have ripe ones every day. Choose them while they are still green and allow them to ripen at home, away from the hands of shoppers in the store. Once ripe, they may be stored in the refrigerator for several days.

BANANAS. Fully ripe bananas are freckled with small, brown spots, and they give slightly when gently squeezed. Bananas do not like to be refrigerated. If they begin to ripen too quickly for you, put peeled whole bananas in a covered container or resealable storage bag and freeze them to make ice cream or smoothies at another time. If you enjoy having bananas in your morning smoothies, you'll need one to three bananas per day per person. You may want to buy them several days or even a week before you need them so they'll have time to ripen. You can also slice ripe bananas into rounds or halves, place them on a flat surface in the sun or in a dehydrator to dry, and eat them as a sweet snack. Another fun way to use ripe bananas is to purée them in the blender and spread the mixture onto dehydrator sheets, with or without added nuts, to make fruit leather.

PEPPERS. Green peppers are unripe fruit, which is why many people have difficulty digesting them. Peppers will not continue to ripen once they are picked, so choose the firmest ripe (red, orange, or yellow) peppers you can find in the market. If you cannot find ripe peppers, choose peppers that have at least some reddish cast to them.

TOMATOES. Most fresh tomatoes sold in supermarkets are firm but not yet ripe. The fruit will ripen properly and develop a good flavor and aroma if kept at room temperature, between 55 and 75 degrees F (13 and 24 degrees C). Select tomatoes at various degrees of ripeness. Fresh tomatoes change texture when they are refrigerated, becoming mushy and losing much of their sweetness, so they are best stored on the kitchen counter away from direct sunlight. Once fully ripe, a tomato can be refrigerated, but only for a few days; any longer than this will result in flavor deterioration. Tomatoes are delicious when dehydrated and used in sauces and dressings.

ADDRESSING GREENS

Of all the plant foods that support good health, dark leafy greens are at the top of the list. The darkest and heartiest leafy greens are often bitter and tough to chew. To digest them more easily, we need to either chew greens well and/or prepare them in ways that make them easier to digest. Blending them in soups or marinating and massaging them can soften their texture and make them more palatable.

Buying and Storing Greens

Buy greens with fresh, crisp, dark green leaves. Treat them gently so as not to bruise them. Put unwashed greens in storage bags that can be sealed. Place the greens in the bag, gently press the air out, and use a twist tie to close the bag. Evert-Fresh brand bags are perfect for storing greens; they keep greens fresh longer than other kinds of plastic bags by as much as five times! (These bags can be found in most natural food stores and are also available from online retailers.) Evert-Fresh disks are also effective. Place the food in the vegetable crisper of the refrigerator along with one disk. In order for the disk to function properly, do not overfill the crisper. Change the disk every three months.

If your vegetable crispers are full and you have to store the greens elsewhere in the refrigerator, keep them on a lower shelf rather than up high, as the upper area is the coldest part of the fridge and the delicate greens may freeze, especially if you have a top-freezer refrigerator.

The commercial greens that are the most popular, are the highest in calcium, protein, and many other nutrients, and last the longest in the refrigerator are broccoli, collard greens, kale, and romaine lettuce. Other greens that are delicious but should be used within a day or two are arugula, baby spinach, bok choy, spring mix, tat soi, and watercress. A few greens that are highly nutritious but are more difficult to find are dandelion greens, mâche (lamb's lettuce), purslane, and sorrel.

WHY BUY ORGANIC?

Organic refers to the way agricultural products are grown and processed. Organic food production is based on a system of farming that maintains and replenishes soil fertility without the use of synthetic pesticides and fertilizers.

If an item is labeled "certified organic," it's been grown in accordance with strict, uniform standards that are verified by independent organizations. Certification typically includes inspections of farm fields and processing facilities, detailed record keeping, and periodic testing of soil and water to ensure that growers and handlers are meeting the standards. Standards vary throughout different locations, but buying certified organically grown produce (or growing your own) is the safest way to ensure that you'll ingest the least amount of toxic residues.

Organically produced foods must meet strict regulations governing all aspects of production. Organic farming is more labor and management intensive than other commercial farming methods, and it also tends to be done on a smaller scale. Because of these factors, organic foods are often more expensive than conventionally produced foods, but their superior quality, safety, and positive effects on the planet make the difference in price well worth the purchase.

Some of the Many Benefits of Eating Organic Foods

- decreased exposure to known carcinogens
- greater variety of heirloom fruits and vegetables
- reduced intake of chemicals and heavy metals
- superior flavor (many top chefs use only organic foods)

When You Can't Buy Certified Organic

If organic fruits and vegetables are not available, wash your produce well, using a mild, biodegradable soap, and rinse it thoroughly. Vegetables that have been waxed or obviously coated with something should be peeled. Peel all root vegetables that have been treated with chemicals or that have had fungicides added to their soil. Fruits and vegetables with thin skins, such as strawberries and tomatoes, are less safe than those with thicker skins; they are also often less flavorful when they are not organic. Choose produce that has the least concentration of pesticide residues, like asparagus, avocados, broccoli, cabbage, eggplant, kiwis, mangoes, onions, pineapple, sweet corn, sweet peas, sweet potatoes, tomatoes, and watermelon. Nonorganic crops that are reported to contain the highest levels of pesticides are apples, carrots, celery, cherries, grapes (imported), kale, lettuce, nectarines, peaches, pears, strawberries, and sweet bell peppers.

According to the not-for-profit Environmental Working Group (EWG), a simulation of thousands of consumers eating high- and low-pesticide diets has shown that, apart from choosing organic produce, people can lower their pesticide exposure by almost 90% by avoiding the most-contaminated fruits and vegetables and eating the least-contaminated ones instead. Eating the 12 most-contaminated fruits and vegetables will expose a person to about 14 pesticides per day, on average. Eating the 12 least-contaminated foods will expose a person to less than 2 pesticides per day.

Note: This produce ranking was developed by analysts at the not-for-profit Environmental Working Group, a research organization dedicated to improving public health and protecting the environment by reducing pollution in air, water, and food. The information is based on the results of nearly 43,000 tests for pesticides on produce collected by the U.S. Department of Agriculture and the U.S. Food and Drug Administration between the years 2000 and 2005. For more information, please visit www.ewg.org.

TAKING ADVANTAGE OF FARMERS' MARKETS

A local farmers' market is a good source of fruits and vegetables that you do not grow yourself. The produce is usually far fresher than what you'll find at the grocery store, since often what is sold at the farmers' market is harvested the day it's brought to market. Not only is the produce reasonably priced, it is usually grown by people who love being farmers.

If you have a dehydrator or a freezer, you can preserve foods at the height of their nutrient value by buying them in bulk and using them when they are no longer in season. Prices, which are often already better than at your local grocery store, are typically 10% lower if you buy items by the case. Frozen corn works well in raw salads, Fresh Corn Tortillas (page 126), and soups. Fresh fruits freeze well and are great in smoothies. You can also dehydrate fruits and use them in smoothies, as sweeteners in desserts, or as snack foods. Don't be afraid to buy flats of berries or figs, even if you don't want to freeze or dehydrate them. It isn't difficult to find ways to use bulk quantities of produce—in fact, it's fun to eat all you want of your favorite foods when they are in season.

Savvy shoppers go to farmers' markets early in the morning to get the best quality. On the other hand, if you're looking for bargain prices, shop just before the market closes or when you see the vendor starting to pack up. Most vendors would rather sell their produce at a low price than haul it back home. Even after being out all day, most foods will still be fresher than those found in the grocery store.

Be aware that not all vendors at a farmers' market are farmers, and many did not personally grow the foods they are selling. There's nothing actually wrong with this food; it's basically the same quality you would find from any "backyard farmer" who is selling premium produce that is freshly harvested.

Don't be afraid to ask vendors about their growing methods. Many will tell you they are not certified organic but use organic methods. Ask what those methods are. Speak up for organics and let growers know that you are committed to supporting sustainable agriculture and only buy organic produce!

SETTING UP AND MANAGING YOUR RAW FOOD KITCHEN

This section includes ways to help you get organized and make a fresh start. You'll find a list of staple foods you need to keep on hand and where to store them, and ideas about storing and ripening fruits and vegetables for optimal health. You'll also learn time-saving tips to make food preparation simpler and faster, and what equipment you'll need.

Clean Out Your Kitchen

Having what you need on hand will greatly increase your chance of succeeding on the Raw Food Revolution Diet. Having everything handy and easy to find will also motivate you to try new recipes and have more fun in the kitchen.

- Even if you've decided to eat simply, you'll need a few items like a good knife, a blender, and possibly a juicer to get started on the raw food path.

- Refer to Foods to Have on Hand (page 71) for a complete list of staples and ingredients you may want to purchase so you can have everything you need to enjoy a wide variety of raw cuisine. In the beginning, if you want to eat more simply, decide which foods you really need and which ones you can wait to purchase later.

- Remove everything you presently have stored in your pantry and put it in another area of the kitchen so you can start fresh. While your pantry is empty, use this opportunity to give it a deep cleaning. This is a good time to do the same thing with the refrigerator.

- Designate a small area of the pantry to keep any "transitional foods"—those that you plan to eliminate from your diet once you have transitioned beyond them. This may include conventional crackers and chips, canned or instant foods, oils that are not cold-pressed, pasta, and other devitalized foods like white flour and white sugar. As soon as you feel emotionally able, give away (or throw away) these or other foods that do not fit with your commitment to reaching your desired weight and achieving optimal health.

- To create more space in your kitchen, store all equipment that isn't used with the Raw Food Revolution Diet in another location or donate it to others. This may include things like deep fryers or electric frying pans.
- Purchase various sizes of mason jars and other glass storage containers for storing foods. Glass keeps foods fresher than plastic.

Change Old Habits to New Favorites

Table 6 contains a few ideas to help in your transition. The column on the left contains foods that you may want to remove from your diet. In the column on the right, we give you some health-promoting foods to try in their place. Oftentimes you can use the seasonings called for in a traditional dish and replace any cooked ingredients with raw foods.

TABLE 6 Replacing old favorites with healthful alternatives

Instead of these . . .	Try these . . .
binders and thickeners	agar, dates, dried fruit, flaxseeds, psyllium husk powder
bouillon or stock	dried mushrooms, miso, vegetable powders
bread	cabbage leaves, lettuce leaves, raw vegetable wraps and tortillas, unleavened sprouted grain bread (see recipes on pages 122–124)
butter or shortening	avocado, coconut oil, extra-virgin olive oil, flaxseed oil
chips	Flax Crackers (page 128) or Garlic-Herb Croutons (page 125)
chocolate	carob, raw cocoa powder
cooked garlic or onion	garlic or onion powder
cooked tomatoes	rehydrated sun-dried tomatoes
cooked vegetables	marinated and/or dehydrated raw vegetables (marinating and dehydrating will soften them and impart a "cooked" flavor)
flour	dried almond pulp (see page 106), ground nuts and seeds
ice cream	frozen bananas or fruit ice creams (see page 220)
meat	ground nuts or seeds, marinated mushrooms
pasta or rice	spiralized zucchini (see page 87) or other vegetables
vinegar	berries, lemon, lime, orange, pineapple, tamarind
white sugar	dates, figs, currants, raisins, other dried fruit; fresh fruit, stevia

FOODS TO HAVE ON HAND

The list on page 72 shows some of the foods you may find handy to have in your kitchen. Use it as a shopping list when stocking your pantry, if you wish. The more unusual ingredients can be found in natural food stores or ordered through online retailers; all of the items can be stored in your pantry unless indicated otherwise.

When purchasing extracts, flavorings, herbs, and spices, buy small amounts so they stay fresh. Herbs and spices can lose their flavor as they age. If you purchase them in bulk, store them in airtight containers.

The following descriptions provide information about foods that may be unfamiliar to you.

AGAVE SYRUP. Agave syrup, or agave nectar, comes from the juice of the agave cactus, the same cactus used to make tequila. It's 90% fructose and doesn't cause blood sugar to rise as quickly as cane sugar, honey, or maple syrup. Agave syrup is mild in flavor and light in color, making it ideal to use in desserts. Choose light agave syrup for a mild flavor and dark agave syrup for a slightly deeper taste, similar to molasses. Be sure to look for raw agave syrup, which means it has not been heated.

BUCKWHEAT GROATS. In spite of the name, buckwheat is not a grain (as are wheat and rice). It is a seed related to rhubarb. Be sure to buy raw hulled buckwheat groats and not toasted groats (which are also called kasha).

CAROB POWDER. Carob powder is made from the sweet fruit found in the pods of the tropical carob tree. It tastes somewhat like chocolate when lightly roasted. Carob can be purchased raw or roasted as a powder and used in place of cocoa. Since carob is slightly sweet and cocoa is very bitter, reduce the amount of sweetener in a recipe by 25% when substituting carob for cocoa.

DATES. Dates are very good to use as a natural sweetener in desserts, dressings, and sauces. Unpitted dates don't require refrigeration if they are stored in a cool pantry. Once the pits are removed, however, store dates in a sealed container in the refrigerator or they will ferment. The recipes in this book call for soft dates, such as honey dates, but any fresh date will suffice. Date pieces are not recommended, since they are often steamed. If dates are very hard and dry, soak them in warm purified water for a few minutes to soften.

EVAPORATED CANE JUICE. Available under the brand names Sucanat and Rapadura (also known as *tapa dulse* in Latin American countries), evaporated cane juice is a concentrated, granulated sweetener. It is not a raw

VEGETABLES	☐ alfalfa sprouts	☐ cilantro	☐ mushrooms (crimini, shiitake)
	☐ avocado	☐ corn	☐ onions
	☐ baby greens or spring mix	☐ cucumber	☐ parsley
	☐ bell peppers (red, orange, & yellow)	☐ garlic	☐ peas (fresh or frozen)
		☐ ginger (fresh)	☐ romaine lettuce
	☐ broccoli	☐ green beans	☐ sugar snap peas
	☐ cabbage	☐ green onions	☐ tomatoes (cherry, globe, heirloom, Roma)
	☐ carrots	☐ herbs (fresh)	
	☐ celery	☐ kale	☐ zucchini
FRUITS	☐ apples	☐ berries (fresh or frozen)	☐ oranges
	☐ bananas	☐ lemons	
DRIED FRUITS AND NATURAL SWEETENERS	☐ agave syrup	☐ dates	☐ raisins
	☐ currants	☐ evaporated cane juice	
GRAINS	☐ buckwheat groats	☐ oat groats	☐ wild rice
	☐ kamut	☐ quinoa	
SEEDS	☐ flaxseeds	☐ sesame seeds (white & black)	☐ sunflower seeds
	☐ hempseeds	☐ sprouting seeds (alfalfa, broccoli, clover, radish, sunflower, wheat)	
	☐ mustard seeds		
	☐ pumpkin seeds		
NUTS AND NUT BUTTERS	☐ almonds	☐ cashews	☐ tahini
	☐ almond butter	☐ hazelnuts	☐ walnuts
	☐ Brazil nuts	☐ pine nuts	
LEGUMES (DRIED)	☐ adzuki beans	☐ lentils	☐ mung beans
SEASONINGS, SPICES, AND DRIED HERBS	☐ almond extract	☐ fennel seeds	☐ poultry seasoning
	☐ basil	☐ garlic	☐ sage
	☐ black pepper	☐ garlic powder	☐ shiitake mushrooms (dried)
	☐ cayenne	☐ Italian seasoning	☐ sun-dried olives
	☐ cinnamon	☐ kelp powder	☐ Thai red curry paste
	☐ cloves	☐ Mexican chili powder	☐ thyme
	☐ coriander	☐ mustard powder	☐ toasted sesame oil
	☐ cumin	☐ nutmeg	☐ vanilla extract
	☐ Dijon mustard	☐ onion powder	☐ white pepper
	☐ dill weed	☐ oregano	
	☐ dulse flakes	☐ paprika	
MISCELLANEOUS	☐ flaxseed oil	☐ olive oil (cold-pressed, extra-virgin)	☐ sea vegetables (arame, hijiki, sea palm, wakame)
	☐ miso (light and dark)		
	☐ nori sheets	☐ probiotic powder (for making cheese)	☐ sesame oil (raw)
	☐ nutritional yeast (Red Star Vegetarian Support Formula)		☐ sun-dried tomatoes
		☐ salt	☐ tamari (unpasteurized)

food, but it nevertheless is used widely by health-conscious cooks. Derived from sugarcane, this sweetener has a light molasses flavor.

FLAXSEEDS AND FLAXSEED MEAL. Flaxseeds are rich in omega-3 fatty acids, an important component of a healthful diet. Flaxseeds are available in two colors: golden and brown. Although either one may be used in recipes, golden flaxseeds are slightly milder in flavor and will not darken light-colored foods the way brown flaxseeds will. One cup (250 mL) of whole flaxseeds makes 1¼ cups (310 mL) of meal when ground. A small spice grinder is the perfect tool for grinding flaxseeds into meal. Small amounts of flaxseeds can be stored in mason jars at room temperature; larger quantities should be stored in the refrigerator. Ground flaxseeds should always be stored in the refrigerator or freezer.

GINGER. Fresh ginger is essential to meals with an Asian flair, and it's a great digestive aid. It's also wonderful in fresh juices, salad dressings, and warm or chilled tea. Fresh ginger may be purchased and stored in bulk, or juiced and frozen in glass jars to defrost as needed. Freeze whole fingers of fresh ginger sealed in small plastic bags. Whole, unpeeled ginger may also be stored in a cool pantry for a few weeks.

GREEN POWDER PRODUCTS. Vegetables of all kinds are now available dried and powdered, which makes them easy to add to smoothies and other foods. Look for organically produced, low-heat dehydrated powders or unpasteurized liquid products. A favorite of many raw food enthusiasts is Vitamineral Green by HealthForce Nutritionals for its variety of green dehydrated ingredients. Store powdered products in a cool pantry, away from light, and unpasteurized liquid products in the refrigerator. Many dehydrated green products can be purchased in natural food stores and from online retailers.

KAMUT. Kamut is an ancient, nutritionally superior grain—a distant relative of our modern, hybridized durum wheat. It's the perfect grain for unbaked sprouted-grain breads.

LEGUMES. For information on sprouting legumes, including adzuki beans, lentils, mung beans, and whole peas, see page 90. You can sprinkle sprouted legumes over salads to increase your protein intake without adding a lot of fat. Store sprouted legumes in the refrigerator.

MISO. Unpasteurized miso, an important component in Japanese cuisine, is a fermented paste, made from legumes and sometimes grains, that contains friendly bacteria. In raw cuisine, it is often used as a salty flavoring.

Miso is not a raw food, since the legumes and grains are cooked before they are cultured, but like yogurt, it is a living food. There are dozens of different types of miso, each with its own distinctive flavor. Dark miso has a deep, salty flavor, while light-colored miso is both slightly sweet and salty. Always keep miso refrigerated.

NUTRITIONAL YEAST. Nutritional yeast is often confused with brewer's yeast, but their flavors and properties differ. Nutritional yeast is cultivated on molasses, while brewer's yeast is grown on malt and is a by-product of beer production. Even though it is not a raw product, nutritional yeast is prized in raw cuisine as much for its cheeselike flavor as for its nutritional value. Be sure to insist on Red Star brand Vegetarian Support Formula nutritional yeast, the only one that contains vitamin B_{12} (along with other B vitamins), making it a valuable food ingredient for vegans.

NUTS AND NUT BUTTERS. Raw nuts and the butters made from them are great additions to the Raw Food Revolution Diet, as they give us a sense of comfort and satisfaction, but since they are high in fat, they should be used judiciously. Almonds, cashews, macadamia nuts, pecans, pine nuts, and walnuts can be used in sweet or savory sauces and dressings. Raw nuts and nut butters should be kept in the refrigerator or freezer to guard against rancidity.

OLIVE OIL. Extra-virgin olive oil, from the first pressing of the olives, contains higher levels of antioxidants (particularly vitamin E and phenols) than secondary pressings because it is less processed. Olive oil is monounsaturated, making it one of the more healthful oils, but the use of any oil should be limited in a weight-loss diet. Olive oils vary greatly in flavor; typically, the darker the oil, the stronger the flavor. Olive oil will thicken if kept in the refrigerator, so a small amount may be kept in a cool pantry for quick access.

SALT. Salts like solar-dried sea salt, crystal salt (such as Himalayan crystal salt), and moist Celtic salt are considered more flavorful than iodized table salt. However, if you choose to use noniodized salt, it's wise to eat sea vegetables daily or take an iodine supplement. All salt should be used sparingly.

SEA VEGETABLES. Besides being delicious, sea vegetables are a great source of trace minerals and iodine. Adults need 150 mcg of iodine each day to meet their health needs. This guideline can be met by $\frac{1}{10}$ teaspoon (0.5 mL) of dried kelp per day, or about ¼ teaspoon (1 mL) every two to three days. Adding a little sprinkle to your salads or putting some in soups and dehydrated goodies is easy and, most of the time, tasteless. So sneak a little in here and there to make sure your iodine needs are met. Dulse is a dehydrated sea leaf that is nice to snack on when you crave something salty. It comes flaked or powdered and is great on top of salads and in raw soups and dressings. Unlike most other sea vegetables, dulse will dissolve in liquids. Nori is a popular sea vegetable used for making sushi. It is available in ready-to-use sheets and can be chopped or crumbled on raw soups and salads. Nori sheets should be stored in a dry place to protect them from moisture.

SEEDS. Raw pumpkin, sunflower, and light brown (unhulled) sesame seeds are high in calcium and add a delightful flavor and texture to many raw food dishes. White (hulled) sesame seeds will not sprout, so be sure to purchase raw, unhulled sesame seeds. Seeds should be stored in a cool place to prevent the fats they contain from becoming rancid.

SHIITAKE MUSHROOMS. Fresh shiitake mushrooms have a delicious, earthy flavor. When purchasing fresh shiitake mushrooms, look for plump, dry specimens that are buff in color. They should be stored in paper bags or perforated plastic bags in the refrigerator. When shopping for dried shiitakes, look for thick caps that appear fairly clean, not sandy. Dried shiitakes can be stored in a cool, dark place and will keep indefinitely. Shiitake mushrooms are safe for people suffering from *Candida albicans*.

SPROUTS. See page 90.

SUN-DRIED TOMATOES. Although sun-dried tomatoes can be found in many stores, you can also dry tomatoes yourself. Slice fresh tomatoes and place them in the sun with a screen covering them to keep out pests, or use a low-temperature dehydrator to dry them (the recommended temperature is 105 degrees F/40 degrees C). Sun-dried tomatoes can also be found packed in oil; however, they are not as convenient to use, as the oil makes it impossible to grind them into a powder. One cup (250 mL) sun-dried tomatoes is equal to 2½–3 ounces (70–85 g) tomato powder.

TAHINI. Raw (not roasted) organic sesame tahini is delicious in dressings, pâtés, and sauces and can be sweetened for use in desserts and dips for fruits. Tahini can also be used as a base for milk with the addition of a sweetener and a little vanilla extract. Raw tahini is usually found packed in jars and can also be purchased in bulk. It should be stored in the refrigerator.

TAMARI. Tamari is not a raw product, but it does contain live bacteria and adds a delicious salty flavor to dressings, sauces, and Asian foods. Wheat-free tamari is made from soybeans and is safe for gluten-sensitive individuals. When purchasing tamari, look for brands that are unpasteurized.

WHEATGRASS JUICE. See page 62.

FOOD STORAGE TIPS

- One of the most important tips to know about storing fresh food is that *fluctuations in temperatures speed spoilage*. Whenever you remove food from the refrigerator, take out only the amount you need and return the rest. That will reduce the amount of degradation that occurs as a result of the product changing temperature. Even a slight change of temperature reduces the shelf life of fresh produce.

- *A full refrigerator will not store all the food at a consistent temperature.* Each part of a refrigerator has a different temperature and humidity factor. The crisper bins are the best for storing greens. Besides offering the best humidity, they keep the greens from being buried under heavier produce, being pushed to the back of the fridge, or freezing on the top shelf.

- *An overfilled refrigerator can freeze the items that touch the sides*, while the center is actually warm. Allow plenty of airflow throughout the space.

- *Group pantry foods of like categories together* in clear glass jars with tight-fitting lids, and label them with the name of the product and the date purchased, using masking tape and a marking pen.

- *Prepared foods stay fresher in glass containers* and are less likely to take on other flavors or transfer odors while they are being stored in the refrigerator or freezer.

- *Prepared foods are best stored in containers that allow the least amount of air touching the product.* When possible, choose containers that are deep rather than shallow.

- When preparing a recipe, *remove the products from the fridge that need to be prepared first*. Remove the more delicate foods, such as fresh herbs and greens, last.

Remember, taking good care of your produce is taking good care of yourself—and you deserve the best!

IDEAS TO SAVE YOU TIME IN THE KITCHEN

In order to maintain the health-promoting Raw Food Revolution Diet, it's important to have plenty of delicious, easy-to-prepare foods on hand. Doing a little prep work ahead of time will substantially cut down on time spent in the kitchen during the workweek, and it will ensure that you will have food ready to eat when you need it. Food preparation may seem like a lot of work at first, but once you become accustomed to thinking ahead and setting some time aside each week to do a few things in advance, it becomes easier.

Do Daily

- Rinse sprouts and soak nuts and seeds in the morning while you are preparing your morning fruit or making a fruit smoothie.
- Rotate your fruit to ensure even ripening, and check your greens (kale, lettuce, spinach, etc.) to see if they need to be refreshed and to make certain you have enough for meals.
- To save time in the morning, make orange juice for smoothies in advance and refrigerate or even freeze it for a few days. The juice will separate and lose some of its vitamin C content, but it will retain most of its flavor.

Do Once a Week, Perhaps on the Weekend

- Buy fresh fruits, vegetables, nuts, and seeds for the coming week. When you return home, wash your vegetables and put them in sealed containers in the refrigerator to ensure longer life and make them more convenient to use when you need them.
- Wash and prepare all vegetables for juice and store them in sealed containers.
- Wash, dry, and prepare all greens and vegetables for salads and store them in sealed containers.
- Chop vegetables for salads and soups twice a week and store them in sealed containers in the refrigerator for quick meals. Do not pre-cut avocados, cucumbers, leafy greens, peppers, or tomatoes, as they need to be added fresh the day they're eaten.
- Make a couple of raw soups and store them in glass jars in the refrigerator. (For recipes, see pages 186–193.)
- Make one or two salad dressings that can be altered using different herbs. (For recipes, see pages 149–155.) For the best results, do not use fragile ingredients, such as cucumbers or fresh peppers, if you expect to keep the dressing in the refrigerator for more than a couple of days. Be cautious when adding hot chiles to dressings, because their heat will become more intense over time.
- If you desire, make a few raw entrées, dehydrated snacks, or desserts. Good choices to make in advance are burgers, dehydrated crackers and cookies, hummus, and marinara sauce for vegetable noodles.

- Make one batch of vegetable or legume pâté. (For recipes, see pages 142–144.)
- Freeze bananas for ice creams and shakes.

Do Occasionally

- Once a month, mince or press garlic cloves, transfer to a jar, cover with olive oil, and store in the refrigerator. The garlic will keep for weeks.
- Make Pesto Sauce (page 162) and freeze it in small jars for convenience. That way, you can buy large quantities of basil in season and have it year-round.

ESSENTIAL KITCHEN TOOLS

A stove and pots and pans for cooking are among the things you will *not* need in your raw food kitchen! In fact, if you plan to eat very simply, you really need very little other than a refrigerator, a blender, good knives, and a cutting board. Here's a list of suggested equipment and supplies to add to a basic kitchen setup. You can also consider the list of optional kitchenware if you want to make more gourmet raw cuisine.

Basic Equipment

- blender: consider a high-powered type, such as a Vita-Mix or Total Blender by Blendtec
- cutting boards: two bamboo boards are recommended, one for garlic and onions and another for fruits and other vegetables
- food processor: Cuisinart and KitchenAid are excellent brands
- garlic press
- grater or shredder
- knife sharpener
- knives: one 8- or 6-inch (20- or 15-cm) chef's knife, one serrated (tomato) knife, and one nonserrated paring knife
- measuring cups: dry and liquid
- measuring spoons
- peeler
- slicers: mandoline or V-slicer, and a spiral slicer (these inexpensive, versatile tools will help you add great variety to the Raw Food Revolution Diet)
- spatulas: different sizes for mixing and spreading

Equipment for Sprouting and Wheatgrass

- bags: cloth mesh
- glass jars: wide-mouth 1-quart (1-L) and 1-gallon (4-L) sizes with lids, for soaking and sprouting, and storage
- screen: plastic mesh cut into squares, for sprouting jars (use rubber bands to hold the screens in place)
- trays: standard cafeteria size, for growing wheatgrass

Optional Kitchenware

- dehydrator (see page 84 for recommendations)
- juicers: citrus and vegetable juicers (see page 86 for recommendations)
- salad spinner
- sushi mat, bamboo
- zester or fine grater

A Word about Water Filters

Pure water is essential. Most public water systems add chlorine and other chemicals to kill potentially harmful bacteria in the water. Unfortunately, this can also destroy some of the friendly bacteria we need to have present in our intestinal tract in order to remain healthy. Use a water distiller, reverse osmosis filter, or a carbon filter that can be changed at regular intervals. Other types of water filters are available that allow some minerals to remain. You can also purchase purified water by the gallon in stores or have it delivered to your home. If you must use unfiltered tap water, you can allow the chlorine to evaporate by placing the water in an open container, covered with a fine mesh to keep insects out. For extra insurance, you might take acidophilus or probiotic capsules daily to help restore the intestinal flora that chlorine destroys.

Food Processors

The food processor is one of the most commonly used pieces of equipment for cutting and preparing whole raw foods, because it's such a great time-saver and cleanup takes only minutes. Use it for chopping vegetables, smoothing sauces, making raw breads, piecrusts, and pâtés, puréeing foods, and even making raw, nondairy ice cream.

Most food processors have several blades and/or disks available for functions such as slicing to a specific thickness, shredding, or grating hard or dry foods. The most frequently used one is the S blade, which is good for chopping and homogenizing foods. While the S blade is designed to function at the bottom of the bowl, the other blades usually attach to the driveshaft using a stem that holds the blade at the top of the bowl.

Most food processors have a feeding tube or chute that holds the food in place while it is being grated, julienned, shredded, or sliced. Vegetables such as carrots and zucchini, which are longer than the feed tube, can be cut to fit the width of the opening and stacked horizontally. When the length of the shred or julienne is not important, you can use the cylindrical feed tube without cutting the vegetables first.

Most food processors have a safety switch that prevents the machine from operating when the lid is not properly closed. The mechanisms vary among brands, so it is important to read the owner's manual to familiarize yourself with the specifics of your food processor.

When using the S blade, it is important to have an appropriate amount of food in the processor bowl. Too much food will not move well in the processor and can overburden the motor. Too little food will spray out and stick to the sides of the bowl rather than circulating with the blade. In most cases, the ideal amount of food will be somewhere just above the top of the plastic center of the blade piece.

If you process liquids and they rise above the top of the tube in the middle of the bowl, they may begin leaking out the rim. Many bowls are marked with a wet-ingredient line to let you know the maximum fill level to prevent this type of leakage.

In general, use the "on" button or lever when homogenizing and blending for several seconds or longer. For chopping, the pulse function is the most effective. Repeatedly flipping or tapping the pulse button or lever creates different-sized pieces and textures quickly. Pulsing can also be useful in the beginning stages of homogenizing. For example, in making Pomodoro Sauce (page 210), you can fill the food processor bowl nearly to capacity with coarsely chopped tomatoes and other ingredients. The pulse function can effectively chop the tomatoes into small pieces before you process them.

A good rubber spatula makes using a food processor much easier and more efficient. Choose a spatula that has one squared corner and one rounded corner. To scrape food from the sides of the bowl, use the squared edge of the spatula in the same manner you would use a squeegee to clean windows. When processing with the S blade, it's more effective to remove the blade before attempting to remove the food with a spatula. Leaving the blade in place makes it more challenging to remove all of the food from the bowl and may damage your spatula tip. If you do want to leave the blade in place, scrape in the direction the blade turns; this will minimize the chance of the spatula getting wedged between the side of the bowl and the blade.

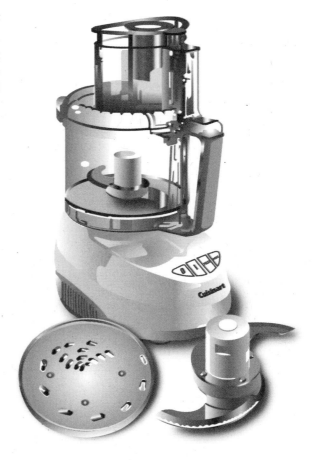

Steps for Using a Food Processor

1. Put the bowl on top of the machine and rotate it into the locked position.

2. Select the blade you wish to use and put it into the food processor.

3. If you are using the S blade, drop it onto the middle shaft and put the food inside the bowl. Fill the bowl only to the recommended level (usually marked on the bowl) or the processor may leak. Then put the lid on the bowl and latch it into place, enabling the machine to operate.

4. If you are slicing or shredding, attach the preferred disk to the stem, drop it onto the middle shaft, put the lid on the bowl, and latch it into place.

Tips for Using a Food Processor

- Trim leaves or other unwanted parts from the foods you wish to chop, and drop them (or stack them) into the machine's feed tube. Push the "on" button, and use the plastic pusher to move the food through the tube.

- To chop food without puréeing it, use the S blade and "pulse" button instead of the "on" button. Keep an eye on the food to ensure the proper consistency.

- Process shelled raw nuts with the S blade to create nut butters. Watch the chopped nuts form a ball, then a thick butter, then a thinner butter. Almonds work well, and cashews, macadamia nuts, pecans, and walnuts also make great nut butters. For ease of digestion, soak and then dehydrate the nuts first.

Warning: Be very careful when handling food processor blades. They can be extremely sharp.

Using Blenders

Always set the blender on a clean, dry, flat surface, and be sure the lid is firmly in place before turning the machine on. Blenders will have a rubber or plastic lid that fits onto the top of the container. Place your hand on top of the lid when blending to ensure that the pitcher stays seated on the motor.

To use any blender, *always put the juiciest foods in first* so the blades can move freely and the juices can draw the other ingredients into the mix. Cut up a few pieces of a juicy ingredient and place them in the bottom of the blender container to start the process.

The lid will have a hole in the center with a plastic cover that can be removed to allow foods to be inserted into the blender while the blades are spinning. High-powered blenders often come with a custom plunger that fits into this hole so that you can push food into the blades without the danger of touching the blades themselves.

Start the blender on low so the food doesn't jump up and hit the lid or spray the sides of the container with pieces of food that will not be included in the processing. This reduces the need to stop the blender, open the lid, and scrape the sides of the pitcher with a spatula. When a proper vortex (or whirlpool) forms in the center of the mixture, you may slowly increase the speed as the food becomes thicker and more manageable; you can then turn the speed up to high without the mixture jumping to the top.

When blending hard foods with liquid to form a purée, add as little liquid as possible at first until the mixture is thick and smooth. Then add the amount of liquid you need to achieve the desired consistency. This will keep the hard food close to the blades, where it can be pulverized effectively.

When creating a thick batter, begin with just enough water to almost cover the ingredients. Start the blender on low and turn it up gradually. When the vortex that forms in the center of the liquid begins to disappear and the mixture no longer moves on its own, remove the lid and use a rubber spatula to carefully lift the top portion of the mixture away from the sides, pulling it toward the center where the vortex will pick it up and move it though the blades. Be mindful during this process to avoid pushing the spatula into the blades or your entire mix (and your spatula) will be ruined. Continue to do this until the mixture is completely smooth and creamy. If the machine begins to lug too much or starts to move around on the counter, add a few tablespoons of water and continue using a rubber spatula until the desired consistency has been achieved.

For easy cleanup, fill the blender container halfway with warm water, add a few drops of dish soap, and blend on a low speed to dislodge the food particles. Use a soft cloth or sponge to clean plastic blender containers, not a brush or plastic scrubber.

Blender Safety Tips

- Never insert a spoon, spatula, or hand into the blender while the blades are moving. (A very cautious exception is described above in the hint for creating a thick batter.)
- Be careful when adding hot food to your blender. Glass pitchers in particular are prone to cracking.
- Don't lift the pitcher off the blender until the motor has stopped.
- Always add liquid when crushing ice. If you crush ice dry, you can damage the container and blades.
- *Always stay with the blender until it has performed its task.*

High-Powered Blenders

A standard home blender will be fine for making the recipes in this book. But if you plan on making the Raw Food Revolution Diet a lifetime commitment, you might consider purchasing a high-powered blender, such as a Vita-Mix or Total Blender by Blendtec. They can blend just about anything in large quantities, quickly and efficiently. High-powered blenders can be used for many of the same tasks as food processors, including making sauces, smoothies, and soups. Unlike food processors, they can crush ice and pulverize flaxseeds, sun-dried tomatoes, and dried shiitake mushrooms into powder. They whip more air into food than food processors—an effect that is desired in some cases and not in others.

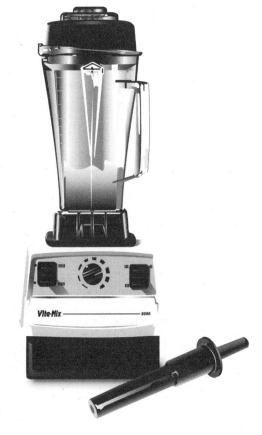

These are no ordinary blenders! They are faster, easier to use, and more powerful than regular blenders, and they are workhorses in the home or commercial kitchen. The Vita-Mix and Total Blender purée and blend more quickly, creating a smoother texture than any regular blender or food processor. Both ensure a perfectly smooth consistency with absolutely no graininess.

One of the best features of a high-powered blender is that it can process a greater volume of ingredients than a food processor or ordinary blender. It also allows you to chop smaller quantities of ingredients, from hard nuts and carrots to soft mushrooms, onions, bell peppers, and tomatoes. In addition, it can be used to make nut butters in small quantities (although you may need to add extra oil).

Another great feature of a high-powered blender is that *most peels, which are usually high in nutrients, do not have to be removed*, with the exception of avocados, banana, guava, mango, melon (except watermelon), papaya, pineapple, and the rinds of citrus. You can liquefy the whole food, including the peel. Foods like garlic and ginger do not need to be peeled before being used!

One drawback of a high-powered blender, especially a Vita-Mix, is that the food can become hot during extended processing. *The blender can actually cook your food!* This is not a problem if you are conscious of that potential and do not process the food for more than one or two minutes at a time. If the food is frozen, it can be processed longer than if the food starts out at room temperature.

Dehydrators

You can make many delicious raw recipes without a dehydrator, but at some point you may decide to purchase one in order to try some of the wonderful recipes in this book that call for it. We recommend an Excalibur dehydrator with 14-inch (36-cm) trays. It has sliding shelves that can be removed, making it very convenient to warm other foods that require more space. There are no holes in the centers of the trays, as with some dehydrators, so you can make a flat of crêpes, crackers, or tortillas without having to work around this gap.

Many gourmet raw dishes require a temperature-controlled dehydrator. As their thermostats cycle, these dehydrators characteristically vary in temperature by several degrees above and below the number you set, so it's important to keep the setting well below 118 degrees F/48 degrees

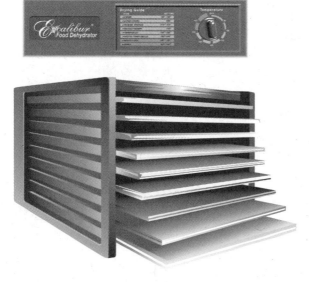

C. However, during the first two hours of dehydrating food with a high water content, you may turn the temperature up as high as 135 degrees F/57 degrees C, provided the food is placed on a moisture barrier like a nonstick dehydrator sheet (which traps some of the moisture inside). The internal temperature of the food remains relatively low while its moisture is being evaporated, in much the same way that perspiration cools us. However, it's necessary to reduce the temperature before the food itself reaches the critical temperature of 118 degrees F/48 degrees C (105 degrees F/40 degrees C is recommended). A good test is to touch the food with your clean fingers; it should be cool to the touch. When it becomes warm to the touch, it's time to reduce the temperature. Food that becomes hot to the touch will not have the same nutritious properties as cooler food; insert a food thermometer into the food to ensure that the internal temperature remains below 118 degrees F/48 degrees C.

A word of warning: A dehydrator can create a bacteria-prone environment if food is left to sweat at a low temperature for several hours and then sits at room temperature. Even food that is free of animal products can harbor bacteria. Gently warm your food for no longer than one to two hours, or dehydrate it fully. If you are interested in achieving a product in between those two states, you must start with the heat high (as described above), turn the food over, then reduce the heat for another hour at most. As soon as the food is ready, place it in the freezer to chill it before moving it to the refrigerator, or serve it immediately.

Here are just a few of the ways we use a dehydrator:

- To speed up the marinating of vegetables. When diced or julienned and marinated in a covered glass container for 1–2 hours in the dehydrator, vegetables soften and obtain a cooked texture and appearance. The dehydrator also intensifies flavors.

- To reduce and thicken sauces. The dehydrator will reduce the volume of liquid placed in an open glass container for 2–3 hours, much like a reduction in traditional cooking.

- To warm food to above body temperature. This creates food that is warming rather than cooling to the body.

- To slow "bake" sprouted breads.

- To create sprouted, seasoned, dehydrated travel snacks like almonds, pumpkin seeds, sunflower seeds, and trail mixes.

- To create fruit leathers, granola bars, onion rings, crispy, crunchy crackers and chips, and more!

Juicers

Blenders and food processors purée and liquefy produce but do not separate the juice from the pulp. In order to do this, you can use them in conjunction with something called a juice bag. Process fruits or vegetables, then pour the liquid slurry into a juice bag and squeeze the bag over a container to catch the juice. This setup will allow to you experiment with the juicing process, but for daily use, you should consider purchasing a good juicer.

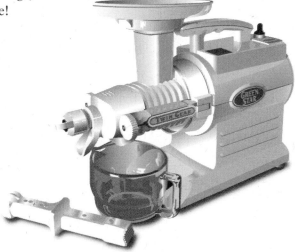

If you are new to juicing and are on a budget, try buying a medium-priced juicer or a good-quality secondhand one. Inexpensive centrifugal juicers wear out quickly and produce low-quality juice with a lower yield, are very loud, and are often difficult to clean. However, any juicer is better than no juicer! Here are a few different types of juicers to consider.

CENTRIFUGAL JUICER. This type of juicer masticates, or chops, the fruit or vegetable and spins it in a stainless steel or plastic basket at a high speed, separating the juice from the pulp. An example is the Acme Juicer.

CENTRIFUGAL JUICER WITH PULP EJECTOR. This machine operates the same way as a centrifugal juicer but ejects the pulp through a side opening. An example is the Juiceman Juicer.

MASTICATING JUICER. This juicer masticates the fruit or vegetable into a paste at high speed and then squeezes the juice through a screen at the bottom. Many masticating juicers can process wheatgrass and leafy greens, which gives them a distinct advantage. The Champion Juicer is a good example.

MASTICATING WITH HYDRAULIC PRESS. This high-speed juicer masticates the fruit or vegetable into a paste, automatically places it in a cotton bag, and hydraulically presses it. An example is the Norwalk Juicer.

TRITURATING OR TWIN GEAR JUICER. This slow-speed juicer causes less oxidation and provides more juice from fruits and vegetables than other common types of juicers. Twin gear juicers will juice grasses and leafy greens. Good examples are Green Star and Green Life Juicers.

Knives and Other Cutting Tools

There are many different kitchen tools that can be used to create a variety of interesting textures in food. Besides the food processor (see page 79) there are graters, knives, mandolines, peelers, and spiral slicers. All are handy and can make raw food more fun to prepare and the dining experience more pleasurable. These tools can help to mimic the appearance and mouthfeel of traditional cooked fare, as well as improve the flavor.

Every kitchen should have at least two different types of knives: a chef's knife and a paring knife. Many people find that a knife with a 5-inch (13-cm) serrated blade is handy for paring thin-skinned fruits, such as juicy tomatoes and ripe peaches, but if you keep your other knives sharp, this knife is not essential.

There are many excellent brands of knives available, and it's well worth purchasing one of good quality, especially a chef's knife, since it's something you'll most likely use every day. Learning to use a knife is important in order to create the desirable shapes and sizes of cuts quickly and safely. It takes practice to become proficient and fast at cutting produce, but even within just a few hours you can gain tremendous skill at this. Set an hour aside when you aren't in a hurry to prepare a meal and use it to julienne and dice several carrots and onions—you'll find it easier to develop your knife skills than you may have thought.

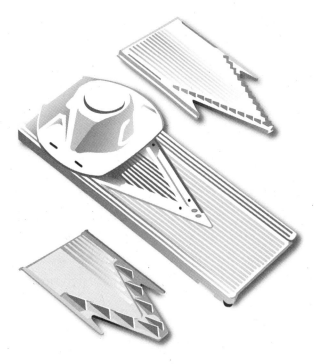

A mandoline is a hand-operated kitchen tool that comes with adjustable blades for quickly and efficiently slicing and julienning firm fruits and vegetables. Mandolines vary in price and function, but they can be purchased inexpensively. This device is extremely sharp, so caution is advised when using it.

A spiral slicer is a handheld device also known as a turning slicer or spiralizer. It creates fine, continuous strands of fruits and vegetables and is invaluable to the raw food chef. A spiralizer can transform root vegetables (such as beets and daikon radish), winter squash (such as butternut and kabocha), and zucchini into strands that can be used like angel hair pasta or linguini. It is so easy to use even a child can operate it, and it's quite affordable.

RAW ON THE GO

After learning about the Raw Food Revolution Diet and seeing its incredible results, many people are concerned about how they'll be able to stick with it when they are away from home. This easy guide will give you the tools you need to make travel in the raw feasible and convenient.

It's completely possible to continue eating raw food no matter where you are or how long you plan to be away. For short trips you'll need a cooler; for longer trips you can create a simple, inexpensive, portable kitchen. Family, friends, business associates, and anyone who happens to be nearby when you open up your portable kitchen will be intrigued to watch you prepare raw dishes right before their eyes in only minutes. They'll be fascinated and filled with questions as you take out your containers and bags holding delicious fresh fruits and veggies, dehydrated goodies, and other treats to nourish your body and spirit. You'll be able to participate in any gatherings and feel perfectly comfortable. Here is all you need.

Raw Food Travel Bag and Picnic Supplies

Foods for Traveling (also see Menu 5, page 98)

- apples (or other firm fruit with skin)
- dehydrated goodies (such as Sweet Nut'ins, page 212)
- dried fruit
- favorite seasonings
- hardy greens, such as romaine lettuce, for salad
- nuts and seeds
- snow peas or peas in the pod

Equipment for Food Preparation

- blender made of lightweight plastic (a small, personal blender with a 1- or 2-cup/250- or 500-mL) container is a good choice if space is limited)
- cloth bag with drawstring for sprouting seeds
- extension cord
- kitchen towel and sponge
- knives (6- to 8-inch/15- to 20-cm chef's knife, small paring knife, and/or serrated knife)
- one or more small containers for cereal or snacks
- one small, leakproof container for salad dressing
- one sealable container for salad
- plastic produce spinning bag for washing salad greens (a specialty item found at natural food stores)
- rubber spatula
- small, flexible-plastic chopping mat
- sealable plastic bags to hold dried fruits, fresh fruits, and veggies

Service Items

- beverage container with watertight lid
- spoon, knife, fork or chopsticks, and cloth napkins (if traveling by plane, pack your metal knife and fork in your checked luggage and carry a small wooden knife and fork in your cooler; some airlines will confiscate your chopsticks, so don't take your favorite pair)
- wooden plate and/or bowl

Other Items to Consider

- chlorine-free water for drinking and food prep (for soups or smoothies and rinsing produce)
- personal water filtration system (especially for travel to third-world or primitive locations)
- placemat or small table cover (a plastic or quick-drying washable table cover is good for picnicking; a lightweight sarong works well for this)
- plastic bags for trash and compost
- soft-sided cooler small enough to meet airline standards if you are traveling by plane
- travel bag for longer trips

TABLE 7 Basic Sprouting

NUTS, SEEDS, OR LEGUMES	METHOD	AMOUNT OF SEEDS PER QUART (1 L) WATER	HOURS TO SOAK	TEMPERATURE IN DEGREES F	TIMES TO RINSE PER DAY	NUMBER OF DAYS TO GROW	GREEN ON FINAL DAY	INCHES READY TO HARVEST	SOME POSSIBLE USES (ALL SUGGESTIONS ARE RAW AND PLANT-BASED)
adzuki beans, chickpeas, lentils, mung beans, whole dried peas	jar	½–1 cup (120–250 mL)	5–10	60–85	2–3	2–4	no	¼–½	entrées, pâtés, salads
alfalfa, clover, radish, mustard	jar	2 tablespoons (30 mL)	6–8	50–85	2–3	5–6	yes	1½–2	garnishes, salads, sandwiches, sushi, wraps
almonds and other nuts	jar	2 cups (500 mL)	8–12	50–85	1	½	no	0	beverages, breads, cheeses, crackers, desserts, dressings, entrées, pâtés, salads, sauces, snacks
broccoli, cabbage, fenugreek, kale	jar	3 tablespoons (45 mL)	6–8	50–85	2–3	3–5	yes	1–1½	juice, salads, soup, sushi, wraps
buckwheat groats in hull, sunflower seeds in hull, winter wheat berries, whole dried peas	sprout in jar, then plant in soil	1½ cups (370 mL)	8–12	50–85	2–3	jar 2–3; soil 5	jar, no; soil, yes	jar ¼–½; soil 6–7	juices, salads, soup
buckwheat groats, hulled	jar	1 cup (250 mL)	8–12	50–85	2–3	1	no	0–⅛	cookies, crackers, granola, salads
cashews	jar	2 cups (500 mL)	2–4	50–85	1	n/a	no	0–⅛	dessert fillings, ice cream, milk/cream, sauces
chia seeds, flaxseeds	bowl	equal parts water/seed	8–12	60–85	n/a	½	no	0–⅛	cookies, crackers, granola, smoothies
onion	jar	4 tablespoons (60 mL)	4–6	60–85	3	6–8	yes	1–1½	garnish, salads
pumpkin (hulled), sesame, sunflower	jar	1½ cups (370 mL)	4–6	60–85	1	N/A	no	0–⅛	cheeses, crackers, drinks, entrées, pâtés, salads, sauces
wild rice	jar	1 cup (250 mL)	24–48	60–85	N/A	24–48	no	when soft and fluffy	pilaf

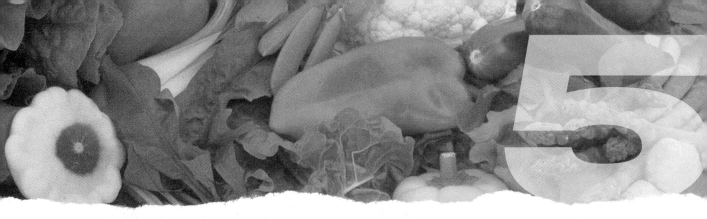

menus to nourish your body and please your palate

The menus that follow will give you an idea of how to use the recipes in this book to create delicious meals that will nourish you throughout the day. Though components of the menus are listed by meal, you may prefer to rearrange them within each menu. For example, you may switch lunch and supper, or eat a particular item as a snack rather than at a meal, or include a snack item at mealtime. Menus 1 through 5 require no special kitchen equipment beyond a blender and food processor. Whereas the other menus are entirely raw, Menu 3 includes cooked foods at one meal. Menu 4 includes sprouted grains. Menu 5 is extremely simple and could be used as a travel menu. Menu 6 requires access to a food dehydrator.

Each menu has been planned so that it meets the day's recommended intakes for nutrients, assuming supplementary sources of vitamins B_{12} and D are included. Below each menu is a nutritional analysis that shows the amounts of calories, protein, key minerals (calcium, iron, and zinc), and omega-3 fatty acids provided by that menu. (Note that optional ingredients in recipes and menus, or ingredients listed as a second choice, are not included in the analysis unless specified.) These can be compared to your exact recommended intakes as outlined in chapter 3. Raw diets are a rich source of vitamins; see page 227–28, for your recommended intakes.

Because this book is intended to help people who want to lose weight, the menus are low in calories, though the food is ample and filling. Feel free to add one or two pieces of fruit or munch on a bowl of raw veggies if you still feel hungry. If you have a dehydrator, try making Spicy Sprouted Lentils (page 217) or Flax Crackers (page 128) to satisfy the urge for a crunchy treat. Chew your food well, as this will promote a sense of satiety and satisfaction. If you want to eat more, you can always increase your activity level, as this will allow you to eat larger portions and still lose weight. Once you've reached your weight-loss goal, you can increase portions or add items to these menus as desired, knowing that your basic nutrient requirements already have been met.

In addition to the juices and smoothies listed here, drink calorie-free beverages such as water or unsweetened herbal teas. We've listed water on the menus to remind you to drink enough. Drinking the recommended amount of water will help you to have more energy and mental clarity and will reduce hunger. Water is an important component of any diet, whether you want to lose weight or not, so make sure you drink between mealtimes and before each meal.

In addition to the foods shown, you'll need to supplement with vitamin B_{12} (see page 52) and get vitamin D in the form of sunlight or a supplement (see page 50). For more about supplements, see page 60.

MENU 1

UPON AWAKENING 12 ounces (370 mL) purified water with lemon

BREAKFAST AND MIDMORNING SNACK A perfect way to start the day is with Green Giant Juice and a Banana-Blueberry Smoothie. Try drinking them at different times so you can have not one, but two breakfasts! This will help to level out your blood sugar over the morning. If you want, you may add any supplements you choose to your smoothie.

2 cups (500 mL) Green Giant Juice (page 119)
2 cups (500 mL) Banana-Blueberry Smoothie (page 102)

LUNCH Try simply delicious Broccoli-Tahini Pâté wrapped in collard or romaine lettuce leaves with chopped tomatoes, sliced red onions, and sprouts. Make one batch of the pâté and enjoy any leftovers served in a variety of ways throughout the week. For example, take sheets of nori, spread them with Broccoli-Tahini Pâté, layer on slivered bell peppers, cucumbers, and sprouts, and roll each one into a log for raw vegan sushi. Slice the logs and serve them on top of a jumbo salad for dinner, or eat the sushi with vegetable sticks for a quick snack.

8–12 ounces (250–370 mL) purified water before lunch
1 serving (½ cup/120 mL) Broccoli-Tahini Pâté (page 144)
1 collard green leaf or romaine lettuce leaves
⅓ large tomato, diced
⅓ cup (80 mL) alfalfa or clover sprouts
1 thin slice red onion

SUPPER Enjoy a garden-fresh pairing of hearty Garden Blend Soup garnished with diced tomatoes and a large salad of crisp greens and colorful vegetables with crunchy lentil sprouts and Savory Seed Dressing or Liquid Gold Dressing.

8–12 ounces (250–370 mL) purified water before supper

2½ cups (620 mL) Garden Blend Soup (page 188) made with sunflower seeds

¼ cup (60 mL) diced tomato

3 cups (750 mL) chopped lettuce

1 cup (250 mL) shredded or diced colorful vegetables (such as carrot, celery, red cabbage, red pepper) arranged on a lettuce salad

3 tablespoons (45 mL) lentil sprouts or mung bean sprouts sprinkled on the salad

¼ cup (60 mL) Savory Seed Dressing (page 153) or Liquid Gold Dressing (page 151)

SNACKS/DESSERT (ANYTIME) No need to give up the simple pleasures of cookies just because you're watching your weight! Figgie Nut'ins are calcium-rich gems that are easy to make and will keep in the fridge or freezer for weeks, ready to eat when you need a quick pick-me-up.

8–12 ounces (250–370 mL) purified water, several times during the day between meals

2 Figgie Nut'ins (page 212)

NUTRIENTS PROVIDED BY MENU 1

Calories: 1,604	Iron: 20 mg
Protein: 63 g	Zinc: 10 mg
Calcium: 1,168 mg	Omega-3 fatty acids: 4 g

MENU 2

This menu does not include Green Giant Juice; instead, it begins the day with a big Blue-Green Smoothie for One that includes banana, blueberries, kale, and oranges.

UPON AWAKENING 12 ounces (370 mL) purified water with lemon

BREAKFAST AND MIDMORNING SNACK Make green your favorite color with this quick and easy smoothie.

24 ounces (750 mL) Blue-Green Smoothie for One (page 103)

LUNCH Delight your senses with creamy Fresh Pea Soup topped with pumpkin seeds and served alongside Kale and Bok Choy Slaw with Spicy Sesame-Ginger Dressing.

8–12 ounces (250–370 mL) purified water before lunch

1¼ cups (310 mL) Fresh Pea Soup (page 187)

2 tablespoons (30 mL) pumpkin seeds sprinkled on top of the soup

1 serving Kale and Bok Choy Slaw with Spicy Sesame-Ginger Dressing (page 176)

SUPPER The flavors of the Mediterranean combine to make this a satisfying meal that anyone can appreciate. Creamy, garlic-scented Zucchini Hummus is an excellent dip for Crudités.

8–12 ounces (250–370 mL) purified water before supper

⅓ cup (80 ml) Zucchini Hummus (page 145)

1 cup (250 mL) Crudités (page 174)

2 cups (500 mL) leafy red or green lettuce

Chopped tomatoes and sliced onions

¼ cup (60 mL) Liquid Gold Dressing (page 151) or Sweet Dijon Dressing (page 148)

SNACKS/DESSERT (ANYTIME) Pure Power Bars, made from figs and nuts, make excellent snacks, whether you're at the office or in the car. They're also great after-school treats for the kids. Fresh orange juice is an energy booster any time of day. Remember to drink water throughout the day, too.

8–12 ounces (250–370 mL) purified water several times during the day between meals

1 serving (2 bars) Pure Power Bars (page 215)

1 cup (250 mL) freshly squeezed orange juice, or 2 navel oranges

NUTRIENTS PROVIDED BY MENU 2

Calories: 1,768

Protein: 58 g

Vitamin B_{12} (from Liquid Gold Dressing): 3.1 mcg

Calcium: 1,010 mg

Iron: 23 mg

Zinc: 13 mg

Omega-3 fatty acids: 7.9 g

Variations

- If you add 16 ounces (500 mL) of Green Giant Juice (page 119) to this menu, you'll further increase your intake of calcium, other minerals, vitamins, and protective antioxidants while only adding 68 calories.

- If you prefer, the Zucchini Hummus can be served on a romaine lettuce leaf "boat" or wrapped in lettuce leaves and topped with chopped tomatoes and sprouts for a lighter meal or snack.

- Instead of serving the Crudités to dip into the hummus, shred or dice them and arrange them on the lettuce salad.

- Those with higher activity levels or who are not trying to lose weight can increase portions or add menu items such as Buckwheat Muesli (page 111), Cinnamon Oatmeal (page 113), or Multi-Grain Cereal (page 112), served with sliced bananas or a serving of Banana Endurance Drink (page 116) for a quick pick-me-up.

MENU 3

This menu is primarily raw; it also includes cooked foods at one meal.

UPON AWAKENING 12 ounces (370 mL) purified water with lemon

BREAKFAST AND MIDMORNING SNACK At first, a green drink may seem like an odd breakfast, but very soon it will become more desirable than coffee! Add several pieces of fruit throughout the morning and you'll have energy to burn.

16 ounces (500 mL) Green Giant Juice (page 119)

2 pieces ripe fruit (such as kiwi, apple, banana, papaya, or pear)

LUNCH If you're feeling challenged trying to stay on a raw diet, especially during the winter months, you may want something cooked at lunch or supper. A cup of warm miso broth or hot bean or lentil soup can warm the tummy and satisfy your desire for hot foods. Beans, peas, and lentils are excellent choices because they add plenty of protein and little fat. (If you purchase prepared foods, choose low-fat items.)

8–12 ounces (250–370 mL) purified water before lunch

1 cup (250 mL) cooked white or black beans (in bean soup, salad, or other low-fat dish)

2 cups (500 mL) steamed kale with ¼ cup (60 mL) Liquid Gold Dressing (page 151), or 2 cups (500 mL) Kale Coleslaw (page 175)

SUPPER Here, the leftover Broccoli-Tahini Pâté from Menu 1 is enjoyed with Crudités and paired with refreshing Apples and Walnuts on Baby

Greens with Poppy Seed Dressing, reminiscent of Waldorf salad. If you prefer, shred or dice the Crudités add them to the salad, then top it with the pâté. Alternatively, enjoy the salad as is and wrap the pâté in a large lettuce leaf with slivered vegetables on top.

> 8–12 ounces (250–370 mL) purified water before supper
>
> 1 serving (½ cup/120 mL) Broccoli-Tahini Pâté (page 144)
>
> 1 cup (250 mL) Crudités (page 174)
>
> 1 serving Apples and Walnuts on Baby Greens with Poppy Seed Dressing (page 179)

SNACKS/DESSERT (ANYTIME) If you look forward to snack time, you'll be happy to know that you can take basic ingredients like bananas, figs, and walnuts and make a delicious pudding in minutes using a blender. Or keep it simple and just eat the bananas and figs without the fuss!

> 8–12 ounces (250–370 mL) purified water several times during the day between meals
>
> 2 tablespoons (30 mL) almonds, pumpkin seeds, or Savory Seasoned Sunflower or Pumpkin Seeds (page 216)
>
> 1 serving Banana-Fig Pudding (page 224), or 4 figs and 1 banana

NUTRIENTS PROVIDED BY MENU 3

Calories: 1,652	Iron: 20 mg
Protein: 63 g	Zinc: 10 mg
Calcium: 1,128 mg	Omega-3 fatty acids: 13.6 g

MENU 4

This protein-rich menu includes a delicious, creamy grain cereal for breakfast. If you like, top it with some fresh fruit.

UPON AWAKENING 12 ounces (370 mL) purified water with lemon

BREAKFAST AND MIDMORNING SNACK

> 16 ounces (500 mL) Green Giant Juice (page 119)
>
> 1 cup (250 mL) Cinnamon Oatmeal (page 113) or Multi-Grain Cereal (page 112)

LUNCH

> 8–12 ounces (250–370 mL) purified water before lunch

⅓ cup (80 mL) Zucchini Hummus (page 145)

Collard leaf or lettuce leaves to wrap the Zucchini Hummus

1 tomato, diced

Thinly sliced red onions

1 cup (250 mL) sprouts

1¼ cups (310 mL) Creamy Kale-Apple Soup (page 186)

SUPPER The longer you eat a raw food diet, the more you'll want just a big, full-meal salad with all the toppings. Use the combination listed below or have 1 serving of Green Garden Salad Bar (page 177).

8–12 ounces (250–370 mL) purified water before supper

1 cup (250 mL) each mixed salad greens, romaine lettuce, and Napa cabbage

¼ cup (60 mL) each lentil or mung bean sprouts and alfalfa sprouts

2 tablespoons (30 mL) each sunflower seeds and pumpkin seeds

2 tablespoons (30 mL) each grated carrot, sliced red pepper, and sliced cucumber

3 or more cherry tomatoes

¼ cup (60 mL) Tahini-Ginger Dressing (page 154) or Liquid Gold Dressing (page 151)

SNACKS/DESSERT (ANYTIME) For a satisfying, sweet snack, treat yourself to Bananas! I Scream (page 220) with raspberry Fruit Coulis (page 222) topped with chopped walnuts. Even easier: eat a banana with ½ cup (120 mL) of berries and 2 walnut halves.

8–12 ounces (250–370 mL) purified water several times during the day between meals

1 banana

½ cup (120 mL) berries

2 walnut halves

NUTRIENTS PROVIDED BY MENU 4

Calories: 1,676

Protein: 68 g

Calcium: 1,020 mg

Iron: 24 mg

Zinc: 10 mg

Omega-3 fatty acids: 2.7 g

variations

- The banana and/or berries from the snack can be served with the Cinnamon Oatmeal at breakfast.
- People who expend more calories can include avocados and olives in the supper salad bar. Alternatively, add a banana with 1 tablespoon (15 mL) of Almond Butter (page 138) and a sprinkle of cayenne.

MENU 5

This menu is ideal on days when you need to cut your preparation to a minimum. The only equipment needed is a blender. It also works for days spent traveling, if you can pack a small mini-blender to make smoothies, soups, and dressings. For simplicity at suppertime, you can blend your dressing, pour it over your salad or into a glass container without washing the blender, and then make the kale soup in the blender. In fact, if you are going to be on the road all day, prepare all your food in the morning. Blend your smoothie first, then, without washing the blender, make your dressing, then your soup. Pour them into separate glass jars and put them in a cooler. Wash your lettuce and veggies, and put them in the cooler too; you'll be set for the day with minimal fuss.

UPON AWAKENING 12 ounces (370 mL) purified water with lemon

BREAKFAST AND MIDMORNING SNACK Breakfast is an important meal and sets the tone for the day—so don't skip it just because you're in a hurry. Make a quick smoothie to hold you over for the entire morning.

24 ounces (750 mL) Blue-Green Smoothie for One (page 103)

LUNCH OR SNACKS ANYTIME DURING THE DAY If you haven't tried snacking on sugar snap peas (also known as pea pods or English peas), you're in for a treat! Carry them around with you while sightseeing or walking during your lunch break instead of sitting down and eating a rich meal. They satisfy that craving for crunchy foods. Other great items for any travel pack are trail mix and oranges.

8–12 ounces (250–370 mL) purified water several times during the day between meals

14 ounces (400 g) sugar snap peas

2 oranges

Trail mix (made with ¼ cup/60 mL pumpkin or sunflower seeds, 3 walnuts, 1 Brazil nut, and 4 dried figs), or 1 serving of either Figgie Nut'ins (page 212), or Pure Power Bars (page 215)

SUPPER When you're too busy to make fancy meals, are busy and pressed for time, or are traveling away from home, it's important to make sure you eat well and keep your immune system strong. Drinking more water than usual is a good idea, and having foods like Creamy Kale-Apple Soup, which is so easy to make yet so comforting, can help keep you on track. Pair the soup with a veggie salad and a simple tahini dressing, and you'll find that food doesn't have to be complicated to be nourishing to the spirit as well as to the body.

8–12 ounces (250–370 mL) purified water before supper

1¼ cups (310 mL) Creamy Kale-Apple Soup (page 186)

3 cups (750 mL) romaine lettuce

1 cup (250 mL) chopped or shredded vegetables (such as carrot, celery, and zucchini)

2 tablespoons (30 mL) raw tahini blended with about 2 tablespoons (30 mL) orange juice and your favorite salty seasoning (dulse, miso, salt, or tamari) to taste

NUTRIENTS PROVIDED BY MENU 5

Calories: 1,658

Protein: 56 g

Calcium: 1,087 mg

Iron: 27 mg

Zinc: 10 mg

Omega-3 fatty acids: 2.2 g

variations

- If you prefer, replace half of the pea pods with 1 cup (250 mL) of broccoli florets.

- Add fresh fruit, cherry tomatoes, or raw corn on the cob (you'll be surprised how delicious it is!) to Menu 5.

MENU 6

If you invest in a dehydrator, you'll be able to add even more great recipes to your raw repertoire. Spend a couple of hours once a week creating crispy, crunchy snacks like Crunchy Buckwheat Granola and Pizza Flax Crackers. Try favorite comfort foods like Zoom Burgers (page 208). Each week make staples such as Sprouted Grain Bread (page 122) or Zucchini-Pepper Wraps (page 130) to have on hand and eat with leftover pâté, diced tomatoes, and other chopped veggies. There are lots of fun dehydrated foods, like Crispy Sweet Onion Rings (page 134), seasoned seeds (page 216), and Falafel Chickpea Nuts (page 218), that make raw meals and simple salads truly special. Here's a tasty menu to get you started.

UPON AWAKENING 12 ounces (370 mL) purified water with lemon

BREAKFAST AND MIDMORNING SNACK Delicious green juice followed by Crunchy Buckwheat Granola, served as a cereal or eaten on the go, gives you a great way to start a perfect day!

> 16 ounces (500 mL) Green Giant Juice (page 119)
>
> 1 serving Crunchy Buckwheat Granola (page 114), as cereal with berries and bananas, made into bars, or eaten by hand as a snack

LUNCH This meal is bursting with Mexican flavor.

> 8–12 ounces (250–370 mL) purified water before lunch
>
> 1 serving Mexican-Style Seasoned Cabbage (page 198) or Mexican Wild Rice (page 200)
>
> 2 Mexican Burritos (page 203)

SUPPER Green soups are a staple for raw food enthusiasts, and it's easy to understand why. They are easy to make, nutritionally balanced, and emotionally satisfying. Add a few crispy, crunchy Pizza Flax Crackers and these may become your favorite at-home meals.

> 8–12 ounces (250–370 mL) purified water before supper
>
> 1¼ cups (310 mL) Garden Blend Soup (page 188) or Creamy Kale-Apple Soup (page 186)
>
> 3 Pizza Flax Crackers (page 129; a variation of Flax Crackers)

SNACKS/DESSERT (ANYTIME) For a protein boost, Spicy Sprouted Lentils can be eaten by the handful or sprinkled on anything you like.

> 8–12 ounces (250–370 mL) purified water several times during the day between meals
>
> ¼ cup (60 mL) Spicy Sprouted Lentils (page 217)
>
> 24 ounces (750 mL) Blue-Green Smoothie for One (page 103)
>
> 2 oranges

NUTRIENTS PROVIDED BY MENU 6

Calories: 1,760	Iron: 23 mg
Protein: 66 g	Zinc: 10 mg
Calcium: 1,021 mg	Omega-3 fatty acids: 5 g

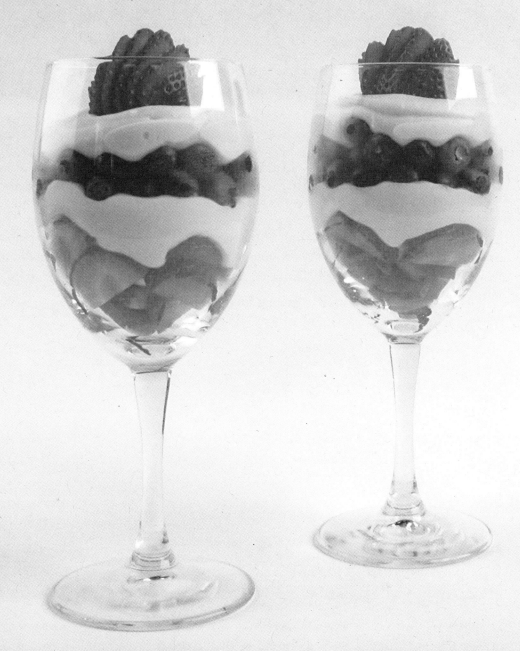

parfaits, using
Cashew Yogurt,
p. 108

BREAKFAST FRUITS AND CEREALS

banana-blueberry smoothie

YIELD: 4 CUPS/1 L (2 SERVINGS)

Bananas and oranges are available year-round, and with the addition of fresh or frozen antioxidant-rich blueberries, omega-3-rich flaxseeds, and nutrient-dense greens, you have the makings of a perfect start to a beautiful day!

4 ripe bananas, chopped

2 oranges, chopped

2 cups (500 mL) fresh or frozen blueberries

1 cup (250 mL) coarsely chopped kale or romaine lettuce (optional)

2 tablespoons (30 mL) green powder supplement (optional)

1 tablespoon (15 mL) ground flaxseeds

Combine all of the ingredients in a blender and process until smooth. Add a small amount of purified water, if needed, to achieve the desired consistency. Serve immediately.

note: Adding the optional kale or lettuce will add minerals and will help to balance the sweetness of the fruit.

a note about flaxseeds

Many raw recipes include flaxseeds. Two varieties of flaxseeds are commonly available—brown and golden. The nutritional profiles are similar, although brown flaxseeds tend to have a slightly higher omega-3 fatty acid content. Brown flaxseeds are more widely available and generally less expensive than golden flaxseeds. However, golden flaxseeds have a pleasant, nutty-buttery flavor, and for culinary purposes, they blend beautifully into recipes without being very noticeable. Either type of flaxseed will work for the recipes in this book, although golden flaxseeds are preferred at the Living Light Culinary Arts Institute.

blue-green smoothie for one

This easy-to-make smoothie for one can be sipped over the course of a morning. If you find the deep blue-green color created by mixing mineral-rich kale and antioxidant-rich blueberries unusual, serve it in a mug rather than a glass.

2–3 cups (500–750 mL) coarsely chopped kale, firmly packed

1¼ cups (310 mL) fresh or frozen blueberries

1 large ripe banana, broken into chunks

1 medium-size orange, coarsely chopped

½–1 cup (120–250 mL) purified water

Combine all of the ingredients in a blender and process until smooth. Add purified water as needed to achieve the desired consistency. Serve immediately.

NUTRITION NOTE A Blue-Green Smoothie delivers 7 grams of protein plus more than 20% of your day's supply of calcium, magnesium, and potassium, and six B vitamins (folate, niacin, pantothenic acid, riboflavin, thiamin, and vitamin B_6). Furthermore, it supplies your recommended intake of vitamins C and K and beta-carotene several times over.

strawberry-peach smoothie

This fabulous smoothie makes a light, refreshing breakfast, lunch, or dessert. The combination of strawberries and peaches is delightful.

2 cups (500 mL) coarsely chopped ripe peaches or nectarines

2 cups (500 mL) fresh or frozen strawberries

2 oranges, coarsely chopped

1 cup (250 mL) coarsely chopped kale or romaine lettuce, firmly packed

2 tablespoons (30 mL) green powder supplement (optional)

Combine all of the ingredients in a blender and process until smooth. Add purified water as needed to facilitate processing and achieve the desired consistency. Serve immediately.

NUTRITION NOTE This smoothie is low in fat and high in antioxidants, and with the addition of greens, its nutrient density soars! With only 206 calories, a single serving packs over 100% of the RDA for vitamins C and K, an impressive 11 grams of fiber, and 142 mg of calcium.

mango-pineapple smoothie

This smoothie combines a colorful and delicious bounty of fruits.

3 ripe bananas, broken into chunks

2 ripe mangoes, peeled and chopped, or 2 ounces (56 g) dried mango, soaked for 1 hour and drained

1 cup (250 mL) coarsely chopped fresh or frozen pineapple

1 cup (250 mL) coarsely chopped kale or romaine lettuce

Combine all of the ingredients in a blender and process until smooth. Add purified water as needed to facilitate processing and achieve the desired consistency. Serve immediately.

NUTRITION NOTE A tropical treat, this smoothie provides good staying power with 346 calories per serving. With the addition of greens, especially kale, you're assured your daily dose of vitamin K and carotenoids. Of course, there's also a respectable amount of vitamin C and calcium. Changing the fruits in smoothies provides interesting variations in nutrients. For example, in this smoothie, bananas boost the vitamin B_6 to 85% of the RDA and potassium to almost 1,200 mg per serving, and pineapple helps to push the manganese to 1.7 mg, or 95% of the RDA.

almond milk

If you like the flavor and creaminess of milk, you'll love this slightly sweet, pure white beverage that mimics the look and taste of its dairy counterpart. In fact, once people taste fresh nut milks, they rarely go back to dairy milk. Play with the sweetness by varying the amount of dates you use, and adjust the thickness by adding more or less water. You'll be pleasantly surprised at the possibilities, as this recipe can be used to create a light refreshing milk or thick, sweet cream.

½ cup (120 mL) whole raw almonds, soaked for 8–12 hours, rinsed, and drained

2 cups (500 mL) purified water

2–3 pitted dates (see note)

¼ teaspoon (1 mL) vanilla extract

1. Combine all of the ingredients in a blender and process until smooth.

2. To separate the milk from the pulp, squeeze the mixture through a cloth mesh bag or a double layer of cheesecloth. Reserve the pulp.

3. Serve at room temperature or chilled. Stored in a sealed glass jar in the refrigerator, Almond Milk will keep for up to 4 days.

variation

ALMOND CREAM: Reduce the water to ½–¾ cup (120–180 mL). Proceed as directed.

notes

- Dates vary in size and degree of sweetness. If you're using larger, sweeter dates, such as Medjool dates, you may wish to use 2 dates rather than 3.

- Store leftover almond pulp in an airtight container in the refrigerator for up to 6 days, or in the freezer for up to 4 months (defrost before using). The pulp may be used in other recipes, or you can dehydrate it and then grind it in a food processor and use it as a flour.

NUTRITION NOTE Remember that this is a nut-based recipe, so keep your serving sizes moderate. You can also increase the water content to reduce the calories per cup. Save the mineral-rich pulp for use in Garlic-Herb Croutons (page 125).

sweet cashew cream

YIELD: 1½ CUPS/370 ML (6 SERVINGS)

This luscious cream is thick, sweet, and perfect for chai. You can also pour it over break-fast cereals, fresh berries, and fruit salads, or serve it as a topping for pies and cakes. You'll never miss dairy cream once you try this!

¼ cup (60 mL) pitted dates, packed, or agave syrup

1 cup (250 mL) cashews, soaked for 2–4 hours, rinsed, and drained

½ cup (120 mL) purified water

1. Loosely separate the dates and place them in a blender with the cashews and water. Process until smooth, adding more water to thin, if necessary.

2. Chill for at least 1 hour before using. Stored in a sealed glass jar in the refrigerator, Sweet Cashew Cream will keep for up to 1 week.

variation: Use less water to create a thick cream for desserts.

NUTRITION NOTE This cream is quite rich, with 10 grams of fat per serving, as it is based on nuts, so use it in moderation. As an unexpected bonus, a single serving of this sweet topping provides 4 grams of protein and over 15% of the RDA for copper, magnesium, manganese, and zinc.

cashew yogurt

Pictured on p. 101

YIELD: 3 CUPS/750 ML (12 SERVINGS)

This dairy-free yogurt is a delicious source of friendly bacteria. It's slightly tart and rich in flavor. Use it as a base for creamy salad dressings, or sweeten it and serve it in a parfait glass between layers of sweet berries.

2 cups (500 mL) cashews, soaked for 2–4 hours, rinsed, and drained

1½ cups (370 mL) purified water

¼ teaspoon (1 mL) probiotic powder (see nutrition note)

1. Combine the cashews, water, and probiotic powder in a blender and process until smooth and creamy. Add more water, if needed, to achieve a smooth texture.

2. Pour the thick cream into a 1-quart (1-L) glass jar and cover the top with cheesecloth. Place it in a warm (65–85 degrees F/18–29 degrees C) location to ferment for 8–12 hours, or until it has fermented to suit your taste. (Less fermentation time is required in warmer weather.)

3. Stored in a sealed glass container in the refrigerator, Cashew Yogurt will keep for up to 1 week.

variations: Other nuts and seeds may also be used to make yogurt, including macadamia nuts, peeled almonds, and sunflower seeds.

NUTRITION NOTE Cashew Yogurt is nut based, so with 10 grams of fat per ¼-cup (60-mL) serving, remember to keep your serving sizes moderate. Health advocates have sung the praises of yogurt as a rich source of healthful bacteria (probiotics) for centuries. Historically, people throughout the world have consumed a variety of fermented foods to provide them with a reliable source of probiotics. Daily intake of foods containing probiotics supports the establishment of friendly bacteria in the intestine. Gastrointestinal tract function may be affected when the delicate balance between "bad" (harmful) and "good" (beneficial) bacteria is upset. Stress, illness, and antibiotics can throw this system out of whack, but probiotics can help restore balance. Experts suggest that probiotics may improve digestion and regularity, increase absorption of minerals, reduce blood cholesterol levels, and protect against tumors.

fresh fruit salad

Fruit salad makes a wonderful base for breakfast—simply top it with sprouted grains, nuts, seeds, and a little nut cream or yogurt. It also makes a perfect replacement for any high-calorie, low-nutrient snack or dessert. Use any fresh fruit combination you like. For an exotic touch, garnish your fruit salad with a sprinkling of pomegranate seeds.

8 cups (2 L; about 2 pounds/900 g) diced ripe fruit (apricots, bananas, mangoes, papaya, peaches, pineapple, and/or strawberries)

½ cup (120 mL) freshly squeezed orange juice

1 cup (250 mL) Cashew Yogurt (page 108; optional)

1. Combine the fruit and orange juice in a large bowl and toss gently.
2. Serve immediately with the optional yogurt.

variations

BANANA-MANGO SALAD: Use 4 bananas, 2 diced mangoes, and 2 cups (500 mL) diced orange segments.

BANANA-APRICOT SALAD: Use 4 bananas, 6 apricots, and 2 cups (500 mL) diced orange segments.

BANANA-BERRY SALAD: Use 4 bananas, 2 cups (500 mL) berries, and 2 cups (500 mL) diced orange segments.

NUTRITION NOTE Fresh, ripe, organically grown seasonal fruit is bursting with vitamins, antioxidants, and a host of protective phytochemicals. Fruit is such an amazing weight-loss ally—it will satisfy your sweet tooth with an incredible medley of flavors and textures, and it contains an impressive supply of fiber.

mangoes in lemon-ginger sauce

YIELD: 2 CUPS/500 ML (2 SERVINGS)

This delightful mango side dish is sweet and tangy, with the warmth of ginger and a high note of lemon. It's the perfect accompaniment to any Asian, Pacific Rim, or Latin American meal. It's also lovely served for brunch on a bed of bitter greens.

2 pitted dates

1 tablespoon (15 mL) freshly squeezed lemon or lime juice

1 teaspoon (5 mL) grated fresh ginger

2 ripe mangoes, diced into 1-inch (2.5-cm) cubes

1. If the dates are very hard and dry, soak them in warm purified water for a few minutes to soften before blending. Drain before using.

2. Combine the dates, lemon juice, and ginger in a blender and add enough purified water to facilitate blending. Process until smooth and creamy.

3. Place the mangoes in a large bowl, pour the blended sauce over them, and toss gently. Serve immediately.

NUTRITION NOTE What is the most commonly consumed fruit in the world? Apples? Bananas? You might be surprised to learn it's mangoes. They top bananas by a factor of 3 to 1 and apples by 10 to 1. Mangoes provide a good supply of carotenoids and vitamin C.

buckwheat muesli

This comforting breakfast cereal can be served in a bowl with bananas, walnuts, and raisins or poured into a glass for breakfast on the go. It can be served gently warmed in the winter months or chilled in summer. Leftovers can be spread onto dehydrator sheets and dried to form crisp, sweet crackers.

¼ cup (60 mL) pitted dates, packed

1¼ cups (310 mL) raw buckwheat groats, soaked and sprouted (see note)

1 cup (250 mL) purified water

¼ cup (60 mL) ground flaxseeds

¼ cup (60 mL) pumpkin seeds, soaked for 4–6 hours, rinsed, and drained

¼ cup (60 mL) sesame seeds, soaked for 4–6 hours, rinsed, and drained

¼ cup (60 mL) sunflower seeds, soaked for 4–6 hours, rinsed, and drained

1½ ripe bananas, sliced

2 tablespoons (30 mL) raisins or currants

2 tablespoons (30 mL) chopped walnuts

½ teaspoon (2 mL) ground cinnamon

1. Loosely separate the dates. If they are very hard and dry, soak them in warm purified water for a few minutes to soften. Drain before using.

2. Place the dates in a blender with the buckwheat, water, flaxseeds, pumpkins seeds, sesame seeds, and sunflower seeds. Process until smooth.

3. To serve, top with the bananas, raisins, and walnuts, and sprinkle with the cinnamon.

4. Stored in an airtight container in the refrigerator, Buckwheat Muesli will keep for up to 1 day.

note: Toasted buckwheat, also known as kasha, is a very popular Middle Eastern grain and can be easily confused with the raw groats. Make sure to buy only raw, hulled buckwheat groats.

To sprout buckwheat groats, first soak them in water to cover for 8–12 hours. Drain and rinse them, and put them in a colander over a plate to catch any water. Allow them to germinate for 12–24 hours, rinsing them every 12 hours. These sprouts do not need to grow tails; in fact, they are better if they are only soaked and allowed to germinate for a short time.

NUTRITION NOTE One serving of this muesli provides 21 grams of protein, 16 grams of fiber, 152 mg of calcium, and over 35% of the RDA for copper, iron, magnesium, manganese, niacin, phosphorus, and thiamin. With 2.8 mg of omega-3 fatty acids and 4.9 mg of omega-6 fatty acids, it also offers an excellent complement of essential fats. Soaking nuts, seeds, and grains helps to increase the availability of their minerals.

multi-grain cereal

This satisfying sprouted cereal is scrumptious served with bananas and raisins or other sweet fruit. It's fun and easy to sprout the grains for this recipe. They take only a couple of days to sprout and can be stored in the refrigerator for several days once they're ready to eat. See page 90 for information on how to sprout.

½ cup (120 mL) pitted dates, packed

1½ cups (370 mL) purified water

¼ cup (60 mL) kamut berries, sprouted 1 day

¼ cup (60 mL) oat groats, sprouted 1 day

¼ cup (60 mL) quinoa, sprouted 1 day

¼ cup (60 mL) buckwheat groats, sprouted 1 day (see note, page 111)

¼ cup (60 mL) sesame seeds, soaked for 4–6 hours, rinsed, and drained

¼ cup (60 mL) sunflower seeds, soaked for 4–6 hours, rinsed, and drained

2 ripe bananas, sliced

¼ cup (60 mL) raisins

½ teaspoon (2 mL) ground cinnamon

1. If the dates are very hard and dry, soak them in warm purified water for a few minutes to soften. Drain before using.

2. Loosely separate the dates and place them in a blender with the water. Process until smooth.

3. Add the sprouted grains and the seeds and process again, adding a little more water as needed to achieve a thick consistency similar to oatmeal.

4. To serve, top with the bananas and raisins and sprinkle with the cinnamon. Enjoy with Almond Milk (page 106), if desired.

5. Stored in an airtight container in the refrigerator, Multi-Grain Cereal will keep for up to 1 day.

NUTRITION NOTE Multi-Grain Cereal provides 595 calories per serving with 15 grams of protein, 15 grams of fiber, and over 25% of the RDA for iron, manganese, potassium, thiamin, and vitamin B$_6$.

cinnamon oatmeal

O ats are one of those comfort foods that remind us of childhood. This porridge goes a step beyond the old-fashioned rolled oats with brown sugar and cream that Grandma used to make. Instead of cooked rolled oats, soaked oat groats are used. Cinnamon Oatmeal is excellent served alone or with warmed Almond Milk (page 106) and apricots or bananas.

1 cup (250 mL) oat groats

½ apple, chopped

2 tablespoons (30 mL) purified water

½ teaspoon (2 mL) ground cinnamon

3 tablespoons (45 mL) raisins

Pinch of salt

1. Soak the oat groats for 8–12 hours in 3 cups (750 mL) of purified water.

2. Drain the groats, rinse, cover again with fresh water, and allow to soak for another 8–12 hours. Drain and rinse the oats once more. Use the groats immediately or store them in a sealed container in the refrigerator for up to 3 days.

3. To make the oatmeal, combine the soaked groats, apple, water, and cinnamon in a food processor fitted with the S blade and process into a coarse porridge. Add the raisins and salt and process for 10 seconds longer. Serve immediately.

NUTRITION NOTE Each serving of Cinnamon Oatmeal provides 387 calories, 12 grams of protein, 9 grams of fiber, and over 50% of the RDA for iron.

crunchy buckwheat granola

REQUIRES A DEHYDRATOR   **YIELD: 3 QUARTS/3 L (6–9 SERVINGS)**

This crispy, crunchy granola cereal is a lifesaver for many raw food enthusiasts. It's delicious with Almond Milk (page 106) or apple juice and sliced bananas, berries, or peaches. Crunchy Buckwheat Granola is easy to make and can be formed into granola bars for tasty travel treats or afternoon snacks.

1 cup (250 mL) pitted dates, packed

½ cup (120 mL) purified water

2½ cups (620 mL) raw buckwheat groats, soaked and sprouted (see note, page 111)

¾ cup (180 mL) currants or raisins

¼ cup (60 mL) flaxseeds, soaked for 8–12 hours in ½ cup (120 mL) purified water (do not rinse or drain)

¼ cup (60 mL) pumpkin seeds, soaked for 4–6 hours, rinsed, and drained

¼ cup (60 mL) sesame seeds, soaked for 4–6 hours, rinsed, and drained

¼ cup (60 mL) sunflower seeds, soaked for 4–6 hours, rinsed, and drained

1 teaspoon (5 mL) ground cinnamon

1. Loosely separate the dates. If the dates are very hard and dry, soak them in warm purified water for a few minutes to soften. Drain before using.

2. Place the dates in a blender with the water and process into a smooth paste. Add more water as necessary to facilitate processing.

3. Combine the buckwheat groats, currants, flaxseeds, pumpkin seeds, sesame seeds, and sunflower seeds in a large bowl. Add the date paste and stir well or mix with your hands to make a batter.

4. Evenly spread 3 cups (750 mL) of the batter no more than ¼ inch (5 mm) thick onto a dehydrator tray lined with a nonstick sheet. Repeat until all of the batter is used.

5. Dehydrate for 8 hours at 105 degrees F/40 degrees C. Flip the granola onto a mesh dehydrator tray and continue dehydrating for 24 hours longer, until completely dry.

5. Break the granola apart or crumble it into chunks.

6. Stored in sealed glass jars in the refrigerator, Crunchy Buckwheat Granola will keep for up to 3 months.

NUTRITION NOTE Crunchy Buckwheat Granola provides a nice complement of vitamins and minerals and almost 9 grams of fiber per serving.

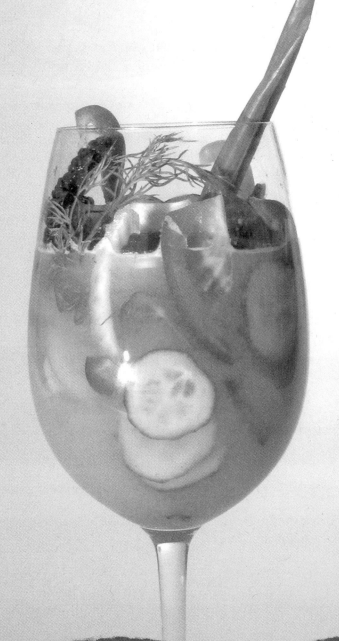

beverages
BEVERAGES AND TONICS

gingery apple-lime cocktail

REQUIRES A JUICER   **YIELD: 3 CUPS/750 ML (2–3 SERVINGS)**

A tantalizing and refreshing balance of sweet-and-tart flavors, this cocktail is a perfect party drink. You can add more or less ginger depending on your preference. It'll satisfy your sweet tooth when you feel a need for dessert. It is especially delightful warmed with a pinch of cinnamon.

4½ pounds (2 kg) apples, quartered

4½ limes, peeled

1 (½-inch/1-cm) piece fresh ginger

Juice all of the ingredients. Serve immediately.

banana endurance drink

YIELD: 4 CUPS/1 L (2 SERVINGS)

M ake this drink thin to sip on while you exercise, or use less water to make it thicker and enjoy it following your exercise.

6 ripe bananas, coarsely broken into chunks

3 stalks celery, coarsely sliced

Combine the bananas and celery in a blender and process until smooth. Add purified water to thin, if desired. Serve immediately.

NUTRITION NOTE Potassium-rich bananas and sodium-rich celery combined with purified water offer the perfect way to replenish your electrolytes and energize muscles following exercise.

cucumber water

Cucumber water is a tremendously refreshing beverage and a great choice for anyone wanting calorie-free refreshment. It's often served in European fine-dining restaurants and is a nice alternative to lemon water.

1 quart (1 L) purified water

¼ cucumber, peeled, seeded, and diced

Combine the water and cucumber in a glass 1-gallon (4-L) jar and refrigerate for 1 hour before serving. Stored in a sealed glass jar in the refrigerator, Cucumber Water will keep for up to 1 day.

variations: Add edible flowers of any kind or a sprig of fresh mint.

ginger blast

With its pungent, delightful flavor, ginger is indispensable in the culinary arts. This sweet-and-spicy ginger beverage will warm and revitalize you. It's particularly pleasant served warm on a cold night, and it's equally welcome served chilled on a summer day.

2½ cups (620 mL) purified water

2 tablespoons (30 mL) agave syrup

1 tablespoon (15 mL) Ginger Juice (see page 182)

Combine the water, agave syrup, and Ginger Juice in a glass jar and stir. Stored in a sealed jar in the refrigerator, Ginger Blast will keep for up to 4 days.

NUTRITION NOTE In ancient China, ginger was regarded as a healing gift from God, and it's still valued today for its warming and healing properties. Ginger boasts a long list of medicinal properties including anti-inflammatory, antioxidant, and antinausea. A sliver of ginger under the tongue has been found to be a more safe and effective motion-sickness suppressor than the most potent motion-sickness drug.

hibiscus cooler

Serve this refreshing aperitif in a wine glass at an elegant dinner party or as a summer afternoon refresher. It's a unique and revitalizing drink that is sweet and full flavored.

1 quart (1 L) purified water

1 orange, juiced (reserve the peels)

½ apple, chopped

¼ cup (60 mL) dried hibiscus flowers

¼ cup (60 mL) coarsely chopped fresh mint

¼ cup (60 mL) coarsely chopped fresh cilantro, packed

¼ cup (60 mL) raisins

4 pitted dates

2 tablespoons (30 mL) agave syrup

2 cloves

1. Combine all of the ingredients, including the orange peels, in a glass 1-gallon (4-L) jar. Cover the jar with a screen and place it in a warm place for 24 hours.

2. Strain and serve at room temperature in wine goblets.

3. Stored in a sealed glass jar in the refrigerator, Hibiscus Cooler will keep for up to 3 days. Remove from the refrigerator a few hours prior to serving to bring it to room temperature.

green giant juice

REQUIRES A JUICER   **YIELD: 3 CUPS/750 ML (2 SERVINGS)**

We love the flavor of this juice and drink it every day.

1 bunch (about 8 ounces/
220 g) kale, including stems

½ head romaine lettuce

1 cucumber, quartered
lengthwise

1 apple

4 stalks celery

1 lemon, peeled

Juice all of the ingredients. Serve immediately.

how to juice kale

Kale is a leafy green vegetable that belongs to the Brassica family, a group of vegetables including cabbage, collards, and Brussels sprouts that have gained recent widespread attention due to their health-promoting, sulfur-containing phytochemicals. It's easy to grow and can even grow in cold temperatures, where a light frost will produce especially sweet kale leaves.

Not all juicers can extract the juice of kale leaves. If you're using a Champion Juicer, roll the leaves tightly and feed them through the chute in small quantities. You may have to put them through the juicer a second time to maximize your yield. If you use a Green Power Juicer, you can extract the juice without having to chop or roll the leaves. Feed the stem end of the leaves in first and allow the twin gears to pull the leaves through without force. Centrifugal juicers are not efficient at juicing greens.

NUTRITION NOTE This powerful, nutrient-dense juice is especially valuable as part of a weight-loss program. It provides 200 mg of calcium per serving, which is as much as ⅔ cup (160 mL) of milk, plus it has 9 grams of protein and less than 1 gram of fat. In fact, the calcium present in kale is twice as available to the body as that in cow's milk!

V-5 juice

REQUIRES A JUICER   YIELD: 3 CUPS/750 ML (2 SERVINGS)

If the power-packed nutrients in this drink don't entice you, the taste surely will!

6 carrots, or 2 apples

1 bunch (about 8 ounces/220 g) kale, spinach, or parsley

1 cucumber, peeled and cut in half lengthwise

2 stalks celery

1 lemon, peeled

Juice all of the ingredients. Serve immediately.

NUTRITION NOTE A great afternoon pick-me-up, this antioxidant cocktail packs well over 100% of the RDA for vitamins A, C, and K. When made with kale, this juice also provides almost one-third of the RDA for calcium.

spicy tomato cocktail

REQUIRES A JUICER   YIELD: 3 CUPS/750 ML (3 SERVINGS)

This spicy tomato cocktail will make your taste buds tingle, setting it miles apart from its commercial counterpart. There are few flavors that better mark the summer months than the sweet taste of a juicy, red, vine-ripened tomato. Although tomatoes are now available year-round, their wonderful qualities are at their peak when they are in season.

6 carrots

4 ripe tomatoes, quartered

1 cucumber, peeled and cut in half lengthwise

2 stalks celery

1 tablespoon (15 mL) chopped red onion

½ clove garlic

2 tablespoons (30 mL) freshly squeezed lemon juice

1 teaspoon (5 mL) grated horseradish

¼ teaspoon (1 mL) salt

Pinch of cayenne

1. Juice the carrots, tomatoes, cucumber, celery, onion, and garlic, and strain.

2. Stir in the lemon juice, horseradish, salt, and cayenne to taste. Serve immediately.

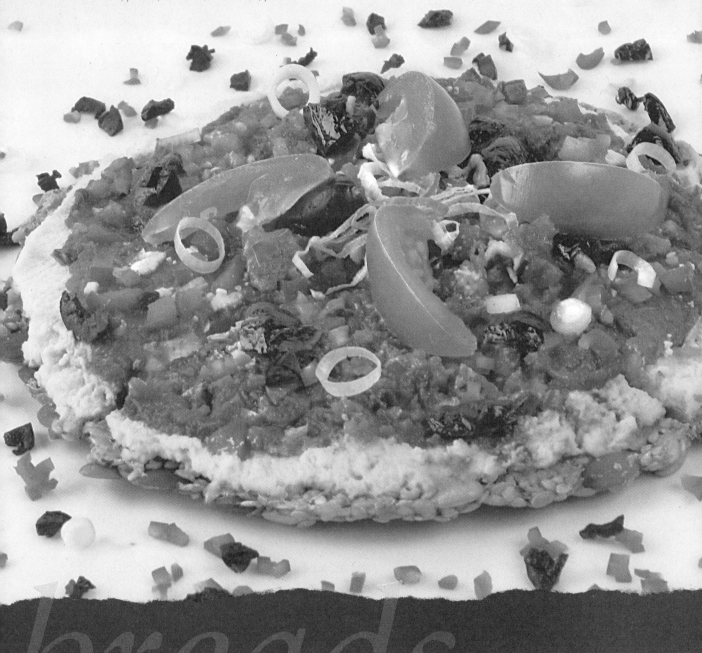

Garden Pizza, p. 202, using Sprouted Seed Pizza Crusts, p. 132,

Pizza Sauce, p. 161, and Almond Cheese, p. 136

BREADS, CRACKERS, CRUSTS, AND WRAPS

breads

sprouted grain bread

REQUIRES A DEHYDRATOR   YIELD: 1 LOAF OR 4 BURGER BUNS (4–8 SERVINGS)

This bread is similar to those made by the Essenes, who lived around the area of the Dead Sea in the time of Jesus. This version is "baked" in a dehydrator instead of on the hot rocks of the desert, but like the ancient bread, it's made from sprouted grain and is unleavened. Sprouted kamut is perfect for this bread, although you may use other grains with equally good results.

1½ cups (370 mL) kamut or winter wheat berries, sprouted for 36 hours, rinsed, and drained

½ cup (120 mL) walnuts, soaked and dehydrated (see page 64)

¼ cup (60 mL) chopped pitted dates, packed

Pinch of salt

1. Process the kamut in a food processor fitted with the S blade until the grains are broken into 3 or more pieces each. The mixture should be sticky but not mushy.

2. Add the remaining ingredients and process into a smooth dough.

3. Transfer the dough to a dehydrator tray lined with a nonstick sheet. Press the dough firmly into a loaf about 1 inch (2.5 cm) thick, or form it into 4 round burger buns, each about 1 inch (2.5 cm) thick.

4. Dehydrate the loaf or buns at 125 degrees F/50 degrees C for 2 hours.

5. Lower the temperature to 105 degrees F/40 degrees C and continue dehydrating for another 3 hours.

6. Turn the loaf or buns over onto a mesh dehydrator tray (without the nonstick sheet) and dehydrate for 2–3 hours longer, or until dry and crusty on the outside and tender and moist on the inside. Serve warm or cold.

7. Stored in an airtight container, Sprouted Grain Bread will keep for up to 1 week in the refrigerator or up to 2 months in the freezer.

note: If you like, the bread may be warmed in the dehydrator at 125 degrees F (50 degrees C) for up to 1 hour before serving.

NUTRITION NOTE Kamut is an ancient grain related to durum wheat; it is higher in protein than wheat and is generally better tolerated by some people with wheat sensitivities, especially when it is sprouted.

sprouted multi-grain bread

I t takes a little practice to get the texture of sprouted, unleavened breads just right, but it's well worth the effort. Once you've mastered the art of raw bread making, you'll reap the rewards!

1 cup (250 mL) kamut or winter wheat berries, sprouted for 36 hours, rinsed, and drained

½ cup (120 mL) rye berries, sprouted for 36 hours, rinsed, and drained

¼ cup (60 mL) millet, soaked for 12 hours, rinsed, and drained

¼ cup (60 mL) flaxseeds, soaked for 12 hours, rinsed, and drained

¼ cup (60 mL) sunflower seeds, soaked for 6 hours, rinsed, and drained

¼ cup (60 mL) pitted dates, coarsely chopped

Pinch of salt

1. Process the kamut, rye, and millet in a food processor fitted with the S blade until the grains are broken into 3 or more pieces each. The mixture should be sticky but not mushy.

2. Add the remaining ingredients and process until well combined.

3. Transfer the dough to a dehydrator tray lined with a nonstick sheet. Press the dough firmly into a loaf about 1 inch (2.5 cm) thick, or shape into 4 round burger buns, each about 1 inch (2.5 cm) thick.

4. Dehydrate the loaf or buns at 125 degrees F/50 degrees C for 2 hours.

5. Lower the temperature to 105 degrees F/40 degrees C and continue dehydrating for another 3 hours.

6. Turn the loaf or buns over onto a mesh dehydrator tray (without the nonstick sheet) and dehydrate for 2–3 hours longer, or until dry and crusty on the outside and tender and moist on the inside. Serve warm or cold.

7. Stored in an airtight container, Sprouted Multi-Grain Bread will keep for up to 1 week in the refrigerator or up to 2 months in the freezer.

note: If you like, the bread may be warmed in the dehydrator at 125 degrees F (50 degrees C) for up to 1 hour before serving.

NUTRITION NOTE The whole grains and seeds in this unleavened bread set it apart from the standard flour-based breads on the supermarket shelves. One serving provides 15 grams of protein and 17 grams of fiber. It also supplies over 10% of the RDA for folate, niacin, riboflavin, and vitamin B_6, over 15% of the RDA for magnesium and potassium, over 20% of the RDA for copper and iron, and over 30% of the RDA for manganese and thiamin.

date and walnut scones

REQUIRES A DEHYDRATOR   **YIELD: 8 SCONES (8 SERVINGS)**

These sweet, dense breads are reminiscent of English scones. Served with Berry-Date Jam (page 169) and Sweet Cashew Cream (page 107), they're truly delectable.

1½ cups (370 mL) kamut or winter wheat berries, sprouted for 36 hours, rinsed, and drained

¾ cup (180 mL) chopped pitted dates, packed

¾ cup (180 mL) walnuts, soaked and dehydrated (see page 64)

1 teaspoon (5 mL) ground cinnamon

Pinch of ground nutmeg

Pinch of salt

1. Process the kamut in a food processor fitted with the S blade until the grains are broken into 3 or more pieces each. The mixture should be sticky but not mushy.

2. Loosely separate the dates and add them to the food processor along with remaining ingredients. Process just until the dates and walnuts are mixed in and broken into pieces. The dough should not be smooth; the date and walnut pieces should still be visible.

3. Transfer the dough to a dehydrator tray lined with a nonstick sheet and press it firmly into a round shape about 1 inch (2.5 cm) thick.

4. Cut the round into 8 equal wedges. Separate them on the nonstick sheet and dehydrate at 125 degrees F/50 degrees C for 2 hours.

5. Lower the temperature to 105 degrees F/40 degrees C and continue dehydrating for another 3 hours.

6. Turn the scones over onto a mesh dehydrator tray (without the nonstick sheet), and dehydrate for 2–3 hours longer, or until dry and crusty on the outside and tender and moist on the inside. Serve warm or cold.

7. Stored in an airtight container, Date and Walnut Scones will keep for up to 1 week in the refrigerator or up to 2 months in the freezer.

note: If you like, the bread may be warmed in the dehydrator at 125 degrees F (50 degrees C) for up to 1 hour before serving.

NUTRITION NOTE With 10 grams of fiber, 7 grams of protein, and a nice complement of vitamins, minerals, and essential fatty acids, these scones are no ordinary sweet treat.

garlic-herb croutons

REQUIRES A DEHYDRATOR　　　　　**YIELD: 2 CUPS/500 ML (8–12 SERVINGS)**

C routons are one of those crispy, crunchy, comforting foods that many raw food enthusiasts miss upon switching to an all-raw diet. This version, made with defatted almond pulp leftover from making Almond Milk, is highly flavored with fresh garlic and Italian herbs, and contains omega-3 fatty acids. They're a perfect topping for your soups and salads, and they also make a great travel snack.

2 cups (500 mL) fresh almond pulp left over from making Almond Milk (page 106)

2 small zucchini, very finely diced

1 cup (250 mL) ground flaxseeds

2 tablespoons (30 mL) extra-virgin olive oil

1 tablespoon (15 mL) nutritional yeast flakes

2 teaspoons (10 mL) minced fresh Italian herbs (basil, marjoram, oregano)

2 teaspoons (10 mL) crushed garlic

½ teaspoon (2 mL) salt

1. Combine all of the ingredients in a large bowl and mix well using your hands to make a soft dough.
2. Place the dough between 2 nonstick dehydrator sheets and roll it out with a rolling pin until it is about ½ inch (1 cm) thick.
3. Cut the dough into ½-inch (1-cm) cubes and transfer them to a mesh dehydrator tray with a spatula (a nonstick sheet is not needed).
4. Dehydrate at 105 degrees F/40 degrees C for 18–24 hours, until dry and crisp.
5. Stored in an airtight container, Garlic-Herb Croutons will keep for up to 1 month in the refrigerator or up to 3 months in the freezer.

fresh corn tortillas

REQUIRES A DEHYDRATOR   YIELD: 12 TORTILLAS (6 SERVINGS)

This recipe, which mimics traditional Mexican tortillas, broadened the world of gourmet raw cuisine, making it possible to create foods like burritos, enchiladas, tacos, and other Mexican specialties without cooking. When these tortillas are fresh and warm from the dehydrator, they're soft and reminiscent of traditional homemade corn tortillas, only much more flavorful. They can also be fully dehydrated until crisp for easy storage, then softened again with a quick dip in water, making them perfect for preparing in advance and keeping on hand. The secret ingredients are psyllium powder and avocado, which keep them pliable yet strong.

4 cups (1 L) chopped yellow bell peppers

3 cups (750 mL) fresh corn kernels

1 cup (250 mL) peeled and chopped zucchini

1½ tablespoons (22 mL) nutritional yeast flakes

1 tablespoon (15 mL) freshly squeezed lemon juice

½ teaspoon (2 mL) salt

1 ripe avocado, coarsely cut into chunks

3 tablespoons (45 mL) psyllium powder or ground flaxseeds

1. Combine the bell peppers, corn, zucchini, nutritional yeast flakes, lemon juice, and salt in a blender and process until smooth. Add the avocado and process until well combined. With the blender running, add the psyllium powder and process for a few seconds longer, until well blended.

2. Using ½ cup (120 mL) of the mixture for each tortilla, use a small metal spatula or flat rubber spatula to quickly form 4 flat disks on a dehydrator tray lined with a nonstick sheet. Each disk should be about 7 inches (18 cm) in diameter, with a little space between each one. Work quickly or the mixture will thicken and become difficult to spread. Continue in this fashion until all of the mixture is used.

3. Dehydrate at 105 degrees F/40 degrees C for 4 hours, or until the tortillas can be easily removed from the nonstick sheets.

4. Turn the tortillas over onto mesh dehydrator trays. Place an additional mesh screen on top of each tray; this will make the tortillas flatter and easier to store. Dehydrate for 3–4 hours longer, or until the tortillas are dry but still flexible.

5. Stored in an airtight container, Fresh Corn Tortillas will keep for up to 2 weeks in the refrigerator or up to 2 months in the freezer.

NUTRITION NOTE Nutritionally, there's no comparison between a traditional tortilla and this fresh version. A single serving of Fresh Corn Tortillas delivers 8 grams of protein, 8 grams of fiber, over 100% of the RDA for riboflavin, thiamin, and vitamins B_6 and C, and over 40% of the RDA for niacin, selenium, and vitamin B_{12}.

salsa wraps *wraps*

Many of our favorite foods are those we can eat with our hands. That makes these tortilla-like wraps fun and delicious! When tomatoes are in abundance, make Salsa Wraps to keep conveniently on hand. They store for months in the freezer and travel without refrigeration for a week or longer.

5 cups (1.25 L) seeded and coarsely chopped ripe tomatoes

3 cups (750 mL) coarsely chopped red bell peppers

2 cups (500 mL) coarsely chopped yellow squash

2 red jalapeño chiles, seeded

1 tablespoon (15 mL) coarsely chopped red onion

2 teaspoons (10 mL) onion powder

1 teaspoon (5 mL) crushed garlic

½ teaspoon (2 mL) salt

1 ripe avocado, coarsely cut into chunks

3 tablespoons (45 mL) psyllium powder

¼ cup (60 mL) chopped fresh cilantro leaves, packed (optional)

1. Combine the tomatoes, bell peppers, yellow squash, chiles, and red onion in a blender and process until smooth. Add the onion powder, garlic, and salt and process until well combined. With the blender running, add the avocado, then the psyllium powder, and process for a few seconds longer.

2. Pulse in the optional cilantro. Do not fully process it; small pieces should remain visible.

3. Using ½ cup (120 mL) of the mixture for each wrap, use a small metal spatula or flat rubber spatula to quickly form 4 flat disks on a dehydrator tray lined with a nonstick sheet. Each disk should be about 7 inches (18 cm) in diameter, with a little space between each one. Work quickly or the mixture will thicken and become difficult to spread. Continue in this fashion until all of the mixture is used.

4. Dehydrate at 105 degrees F/40 degrees C for about 4 hours, or until the wraps can be easily removed from the nonstick sheets.

5. Turn the wraps over onto mesh dehydrator trays. Place an additional mesh screen on top of each tray; this will make the wraps flatter and easier to store. Dehydrate for 3–4 hours longer, or until the wraps are dry but still flexible.

6. Stored in an airtight container, Salsa Wraps will keep for up to 1 month in the refrigerator or up to 3 months in the freezer.

NUTRITION NOTE It is hard to imagine wraps that pack a better antioxidant punch—these are brimming with carotenoids, selenium, and vitamin C. As an added bonus, two Salsa Wraps (one serving) provide 96% of the RDA for chromium—a nutrient that's not easy to come by.

flax crackers

REQUIRES A DEHYDRATOR   YIELD: ABOUT 100 CRACKERS (5 CRACKERS PER SERVING)

These nutritious, crispy, crunchy dehydrated crackers are rich in essential omega-3 fatty acids. They will help satisfy the urge for high-fat, low-fiber snacks like potato chips and commercial crackers. Use sweet red, orange, or yellow bell peppers or ripe, red tomatoes to make these crackers colorful and naturally delicious. They are fantastic by themselves or served with guacamole or raw, nondairy cheese spreads. For maximum use of the dehydrator and to save energy, double the recipe. Alternatively, for a smaller yield, you can cut the recipe in half.

4 cups (1 L) chopped bell peppers or seeded ripe tomatoes

1½ cups (370 mL) peeled and chopped zucchini

½ cup (120 mL) diced red onion

1 tablespoon (15 mL) evaporated cane juice

1 tablespoon (15 mL) freshly squeezed lemon juice

2–3 cloves garlic

1 teaspoon (5 mL) salt

1 cup (250 mL) whole flaxseeds, soaked for 8–12 hours in 2 cups (500 mL) purified water (do not rinse or drain)

1¼ cups (310 mL) ground flaxseeds

1. Combine the bell peppers, zucchini, onion, evaporated cane juice, lemon juice, garlic, and salt in a blender and process until completely smooth.

2. Transfer to a large bowl and stir in the whole flaxseeds and their soaking liquid.

3. Sprinkle the ground flaxseeds over the top and stir well. Allow to sit for 30 minutes at room temperature.

4. Place 2½ cups (620 mL) of the mixture on each dehydrator tray lined with a nonstick sheet. Evenly spread the mixture using a medium-size metal spatula or flat rubber spatula. Score into 6 equal strips, then cross-score from corner to corner. Continue cutting strips parallel to the cross strip, creating 5 evenly spaced strips on each side of the cross-score to form a total of 10 strips. You will then have 40 parallelogram-shaped crackers on each tray (if you are using a dehydrator with 13½-inch/34-cm-square trays).

5. Dehydrate for about 12 hours at 105 degrees F/40 degrees C, until the top is thoroughly dry, then turn the crackers over onto mesh dehydrator trays (without the nonstick sheets). This can be done easily by placing a mesh dehydrator tray on top of the crackers and turning the pair of trays together. If the score marks are no longer visible, cut with scissors where the score marks should be. Continue dehydrating for 8–12 hours or longer, until completely crisp. Break into crackers along the score lines.

6. Stored in an airtight container in a cool dark place, Flax Crackers will keep for up to 3 months.

variations

GOLDEN PEPPER AND SESAME FLAX SHARDS: Use yellow bell peppers and add 3 tablespoons (45 mL) black or brown sesame seeds along with the soaked flaxseeds.

PIZZA FLAX CRACKERS: Add ¾ cup (180 mL) Sun-Dried Tomato Powder (see sidebar) and 1 teaspoon (5 mL) Italian seasoning and blend with the other ingredients in step 1. Add ¼ cup (60 mL) minced fresh herbs (such as basil, marjoram, oregano, or thyme) along with the soaked flaxseeds.

RED HOT CHIPS: Add ½ cup (120 mL) chopped fresh basil leaves (firmly packed), 1 teaspoon (5 mL) chili powder, and ¼ teaspoon (1 mL) cayenne and blend with the other ingredients in step 1.

Sun-Dried Tomato Powder and Purée

Sun-dried tomatoes must be very dry in order to turn them into powder. Moist or even slightly moist tomatoes will not work. Using a high-powered blender, process the dried tomatoes and grind them to a fine powder.

If you don't have a high-powered blender, use a standard blender to make Sun-Dried Tomato Purée to flavor and thicken recipes. Soak ½ cup (120 mL) sun-dried tomatoes in ⅓ cup (80 mL) purified water for 1 hour, until soft. Drain, transfer to a blender, and process until smooth. Use to replace ⅓ cup (80 mL) of Sun-Dried Tomato Powder in recipes.

NUTRITION NOTE With less than 50 calories per serving, Flax Crackers are a good low-cal snack. They also boast a wonderful range of carotenoids, minerals, vitamins, and immune-boosting antioxidants; over 10% of the RDA for copper, folate, magnesium, manganese, and vitamin B₆; and close to 10% of the RDA for zinc.

zucchini-pepper wraps

REQUIRES A DEHYDRATOR   YIELD: 12 WRAPS (6 SERVINGS)

These versatile, disk-shaped, vegetable-based flatbreads are very similar to tortillas. They're great when you're craving something to wrap your hands around. They travel well, so stuff them with pâté or guacamole and shredded vegetables, or sliced avocado, diced tomato, and sprouts, for a nutritious, filling meal on the go.

6 cups (1.5 L) chopped yellow bell peppers

6 cups (1.5 L) chopped zucchini

1 ripe avocado, coarsely cut into chunks

1½ tablespoons (22 mL) nutritional yeast flakes (optional)

½ teaspoon (2 mL) salt

3 tablespoons (45 mL) psyllium powder

1. Combine the bell peppers and zucchini in a blender and process until smooth. Add the avocado, the optional nutritional yeast flakes, and the salt and process until well combined. With the blender running, add the psyllium powder and process for a few seconds longer.

2. Pour ½ cup (120 mL) of the batter onto each of the 4 corners of a dehydrator tray lined with a nonstick sheet. Using a small metal spatula or flat rubber spatula, form 4 flat disks. Each disk should be about 7 inches (18 cm) in diameter, with a little space between each one. Work quickly or the mixture will thicken and become difficult to spread.

3. Dehydrate at 105 degrees F/40 degrees C for about 4 hours, or until the wraps can be easily removed from the nonstick sheets.

4. Turn the wraps over onto mesh dehydrator trays. Place an additional mesh screen on top of each tray; this will make the wraps flatter and easier to store. Dehydrate for 3–4 hours longer, until dry but still flexible.

5. Stored in an airtight container, Zucchini-Pepper Wraps will keep for up to 2 weeks in the refrigerator or up to 2 months in the freezer.

NUTRITION NOTE Prepared with nutritional yeast, Zucchini-Pepper Wraps are bursting with B vitamins, including over one-third of the RDA for vitamin B_{12}. Psyllium is a rich source of selenium, raising the content of these wraps to over 50% of the RDA. As an added bonus, a serving provides over 20% of the RDA for a variety of minerals, including copper, molybdenum, potassium, and iron.

zucchini pizza crusts

REQUIRES A DEHYDRATOR   YIELD: 12 INDIVIDUAL PIZZA CRUSTS

Zucchini makes a simple, bland crust that is fat free, easy to digest, and works well with various toppings. And because each crust contains two dehydrated zucchini, it's very filling. Drink plenty of water with this crust and you will feel satiated in no time.

26 cups (6 L) shredded zucchini (20–24 medium-size zucchini)

1. Cut the zucchini into long, thin strips resembling linguini. A spiral slicer is perfect for this application, but a medium shredding disk on a food processor or hand grater is adequate. If you're an expert with a knife, it can also be accomplished by hand.

2. Place 2 cups (500 mL) of the shredded zucchini in each of the 4 corners of a dehydrator tray lined with a nonstick sheet and gently press the zucchini to form it into 4 round crusts, each about 1 inch (2.5 cm) thick in the middle and 1¼ inches (3 cm) thick around the edges. Repeat this step, forming 4 crusts on each of 3 trays to make a total of 12 crusts. Reserve the remaining zucchini to patch any holes that develop during the dehydrating process.

3. Dehydrate at 125 degrees F/50 degrees C for 2 hours.

4. Lower the temperature to 105 degrees F/40 degrees C and dehydrate for 18–24 hours longer, or until crisp. Use the reserved zucchini to fill the holes that develop as the crusts dehydrate.

5. Stored in an airtight container at room temperature, Zucchini Pizza Crusts will keep for up to 2 months.

NUTRITION NOTE With fewer than 50 calories per serving, this crust lends itself well to weight-loss diets, because it allows you to enjoy pizza without grains or added fat.

sprouted seed pizza crusts

REQUIRES A DEHYDRATOR *Pictured on p. 121*   **YIELD: 10 SMALL, INDIVIDUAL PIZZA CRUSTS**

Sprouted seeds are the base of these versatile, individual pizza crusts, which can be used in a variety of ways. Create traditional Italian pizzas with red Pizza Sauce (page 161) or Pesto Sauce (page 162), or omit the vegetables and savory flavorings and add dates to form sweet crusts for fun fruit pizzas.

½ cup (120 mL) sunflower seeds

1 large stalk celery, chopped

3 tablespoons (45 mL) purified water

1 green onion, chopped

½ teaspoon (2 mL) salt

1 clove garlic, minced

¼ cup (60 mL) parsley sprigs, packed

1½ teaspoons (7 mL) dulse flakes

½ cup (120 mL) pumpkin seeds, soaked for 4–6 hours, rinsed, and drained

½ cup (120 mL) sesame seeds, soaked for 4–6 hours, rinsed, and drained

½ cup (120 mL) sunflower seeds, soaked for 4–6 hours, rinsed, and drained

½ cup (120 mL) flaxseeds, soaked in 1 cup (250 mL) purified water for 4–6 hours (do not rinse or drain)

3 tablespoons (45 mL) ground flaxseeds

1. Place the unsoaked sunflower seeds in a food processor fitted with the S blade and grind them into a fine powder. Transfer to a small bowl and set aside.

2. Combine the celery, water, green onion, salt, and garlic in the same food processor and process until smooth.

3. Add the parsley and dulse and pulse briefly just to mix; flecks of parsley should still be visible. Leave this mixture in the food processor.

4. Add the rinsed and drained pumpkin, sesame, and sunflower seeds to the food processor and pulse into a coarse meal.

5. Transfer the mixture to a large bowl. Add the soaked flaxseeds and their soaking water and mix well.

6. Sprinkle the ground flaxseeds and reserved ground sunflower seeds over the mixture and knead well to make a smooth, lump-free dough. Allow the dough to rest for 20 minutes.

7. Form 4 crusts at a time, using ⅓ cup (80 mL) of the mixture for each crust, and place them evenly in the 4 corners of a dehydrator tray lined with a nonstick sheet. Using a small metal spatula or flat rubber spatula, form flat, evenly shaped disks about 5½ inches (12 cm) in diameter, with a little space between each one.

8. Dehydrate for 8–10 hours at 115 degrees F/45 degrees C. Invert the crusts onto a mesh dehydrator tray, remove the nonstick sheet by peeling it back, and continue dehydrating for 8–10 hours or longer, until the crusts are completely dry and crisp.

9. Stored in an airtight container, Sprouted Seed Pizza Crusts will keep for up to 1 month in the refrigerator or up to 3 months in the freezer.

NUTRITION NOTE The sprouted seeds in these crusts make their nutritional profile something to sing about. Imagine one serving of pizza crust chalking up 9 grams of protein, 6 grams of fiber, almost 60% of the RDA for vitamin K, over 25% of the RDA for copper, magnesium, manganese, phosphorus, and thiamin, 18% of the RDA for iron, and over 10% of the RDA for folate and zinc!

crispy sweet onion rings

Onions are treasured for the sweet and pungent flavor they add to so many recipes. Crispy Sweet Onion Rings are great to keep on hand, as they'll quash a fast-food craving and are great on top of burgers, croquettes, and salads, or as a snack in place of popcorn. Bet you can't eat just one!

2½ pounds (1.1 kg) sweet onions, sliced into ¼-inch (5-mm) rings

½ cup (120 mL) salt (yes, this amount is correct)

2 tablespoons (30 mL) freshly squeezed lemon juice

1½ oranges, chopped

½ cup (120 mL) sesame seeds

¼ cup (60 mL) purified water

1 small pitted date

Pinch of salt

1. Separate the onions into individual rings in a large bowl and cover them with purified water. Add the ½ cup (120 mL) salt and the lemon juice and let the onions soak for 1–2 hours to soften and remove some of their strong juice.

2. Drain the onions and rinse well with purified water, then drain again. Transfer the onions to a dry towel and allow them to sit for a few minutes while you make the batter.

3. Combine the oranges, sesame seeds, water, date, and pinch of salt in a blender and process into a thick batter.

4. Pour half of the batter over the onions in the bowl and toss until they are evenly coated. Arrange the onions evenly on dehydrator trays lined with nonstick sheets, using about 2 cups (500 mL) of onions for each tray.

5. Dehydrate at 105 degrees F/40 degrees C for 6–8 hours. Turn the onions over and drizzle the remaining batter over the top. Continue dehydrating until completely crisp, about 12–18 hours longer.

6. Stored in an airtight container, Crispy Sweet Onion Rings will keep for several weeks at room temperature or for 3 months or longer in the refrigerator.

variation

CRISPY SWEET ONION CRACKERS: Dice and soak the onions instead of slicing them, and add ¼ cup (60 mL) ground flaxseeds to the batter in step 3. Proceed with the recipe through step 3, then pour all of the batter over the onions in the bowl, toss, and spread 2½ cups (620 mL) of the mixture evenly on a dehydrator tray lined with a nonstick sheet. Score into 6 rows across and 8 rows down to form 48 rectangular crackers. Repeat using the remaining 2½ cups (620 mL) of batter. Dehydrate at 105 degrees F/40 degrees C for 8–10 hours. Turn the crackers over and continue dehydrating for about 24 hours longer, until completely dry and crisp. Break into crackers along the score lines.

NUTRITION NOTE Onions are an excellent source of antioxidants. They also have antiviral and antihistamine properties and are high in sulfur, the "beauty mineral."

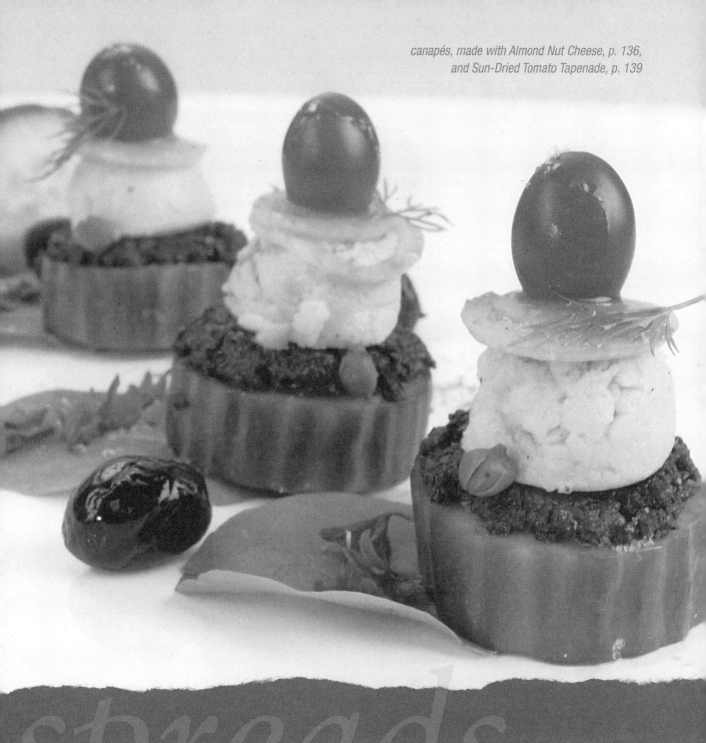

canapés, made with Almond Nut Cheese, p. 136,
and Sun-Dried Tomato Tapenade, p. 139

spreads

SPREADS AND DIPS

basic nut cheese

Pictured on p. 135

YIELD: 2 CUPS/500 ML (8 SERVINGS)

Nut cheeses are as luscious and satisfying as any dairy cheese, and moderate amounts can help satisfy your hunger as you become accustomed to a new, lighter way of eating. Once you learn to make nut cheese, you're free to create foods like cheese spreads, enchiladas, and all the other foods that are just not the same without cheese. Now there are no limits!

Almonds make great ricotta and feta, macadamia nuts are wonderful for ricotta and mozzarella, cashews make perfect cream cheese and frosting, pine nuts are ideal for Parmesan, and hazelnuts are a great choice for dessert fillings, especially paired with chocolate. Have fun!

2 cups (500 mL) almonds (peeled), cashews, macadamia nuts, or pine nuts (see variations)

1 cup (250 mL) purified water

½ teaspoon (2 mL) probiotic powder

1. Combine the nuts, water, and probiotic powder in a blender and process until smooth. Add a small amount of additional water, if necessary, to facilitate processing. However, use as little water as possible to achieve a thick, creamy consistency.

2. Select a pint-size (500 mL) or larger strainer (a plastic berry basket works well) and line it with cheesecloth, allowing several inches of the cloth to drape down around the sides. Set the strainer on top of a shallow baking dish and pour the nut batter into the cheesecloth. The baking dish will catch the liquid as it drains from the cheese. Fold the excess cheesecloth over the top of the cheese, and place the bundle in a warm (65–85 degrees F/18–29 degrees C) location to ferment for 8–12 hours. (Less fermentation time is required in warmer weather.)

3. After about 2 hours of fermenting, place a weight (such as a cup of grain or seeds) on top of the cheese to press out the excess liquid.

4. After the cheese has fermented to suit your taste, use it in any recipe calling for nut cheese. Stored in a sealed glass container in the refrigerator, Basic Nut Cheese will keep for up to 1 week.

variations

ALMOND CHEESE: Soak whole raw almonds in nearly boiling purified water for 5 minutes, drain, and remove the skins using your fingers. Immediately plunge the skinned almonds into cold water and soak them for 8–12 hours. Rinse, drain, and blend as directed.

CASHEW OR PINE NUT CHEESE: Use unsoaked nuts if you have a high-powered blender. Otherwise, soak cashews or pine nuts for 2 hours, rinse, and drain. Blend as directed. No cheesecloth is required, since these nuts will not release any liquid during fermentation. Pour the mixture into a bowl (rather than a strainer) for step 2.

CHUNKY CHEESE: Mix into the finished cheese (at step 4) chopped seeds or nuts of your choice.

HERB CHEESE: Mix into the finished cheese (at step 4) minced fresh herbs, garlic, scallions, and/or other seasonings to taste. This variation may be used with any of the other cheese variations.

MACADAMIA CHEESE: Use unsoaked nuts if you have a high-powered blender. Otherwise, soak macadamia nuts for 6 hours, rinse, and drain. Blend as directed.

MISO NUT CHEESE: Omit the probiotic powder and use 1 teaspoon (5 mL) of light miso as a starter. Blend as directed.

PINE NUT PARMESAN: Combine 8 ounces (220 g) pine nuts, ¾ cup (180 mL) water, 1 teaspoon (5 mL) salt, and ¼ teaspoon (1 mL) probiotic powder in a blender and process into a smooth cream. Spread the cream thinly on a dehydrator tray lined with a nonstick sheet and dehydrate at 105 degrees F/40 degrees C for 12 hours, until completely dry and crisp. Break the cheese apart with your hands and sprinkle it on salads and pasta.

NUTRITION NOTE Remember that nuts are high in fat and calories, so it's important that these cheeses be used in moderation or only as an occasional treat. The nutrient contribution of nut cheeses varies considerably depending on the nuts used. Per serving, Almond Cheese delivers almost 80% of the RDA for vitamin E and over 100 mg of calcium, Cashew Cheese supplies one-third of the RDA for zinc, Macadamia Cheese offers over 75% of the RDA for manganese, and Pine Nut Cheese has almost 3 mg of iron.

almond butter

Making your own nut butter is fast, easy, and economical. If you soak and dehydrate the nuts first, as recommended in the recipe, the butter won't separate and cause the oils to float to the top. Use Almond Butter in place of peanut butter for sandwiches or as a spread on bananas or celery. It can also be added to sauces.

3 cups (750 mL) almonds, soaked and dehydrated (see page 64)

Pinch of salt (optional)

1. Place the almonds and the optional salt in a food processor fitted with the S blade and process for 5–15 minutes, stopping frequently to scrape down the sides of the work bowl as needed, until the almonds have turned into a paste. Alternatively, process the almonds through a Champion or Green Star Juicer fitted with the homogenizing plate, and stir in the optional salt.

2. Stored in a sealed glass jar in the refrigerator, Almond Butter will keep for up to 1 month.

NUTRITION NOTE Almond Butter is far more health-promoting than most nut butters available on grocery store shelves. Soaking the nuts reduces phytates, thus increasing mineral absorption from the nuts. One serving (2 tablespoons/30 mL) of Almond Butter provides almost 86 mg of calcium and over 40% of the RDA for vitamin E—a nutrient that most people fall short on. By contrast, the same size serving of peanut butter provides only 14 mg of calcium and less than 20% of the RDA for vitamin E.

salsa fresca

When Cherie was growing up in California, her Mexican-American relatives used to make this fresh tomato salsa daily and put it on everything. It is quick and easy to make, is fat free, and lasts for several days in the fridge, so go ahead, make a triple batch. Enjoy it served with guacamole, sprouts, and Fresh Corn Tortillas (page 126), Salsa Wraps (page 127), or Flax Crackers (page 128).

2 Roma tomatoes, seeded and finely diced

1 green onion, thinly sliced

1 tablespoon (15 mL) minced fresh cilantro

½ serrano chile, minced, or pinch of cayenne

1 small clove garlic, crushed

¼ teaspoon (1 mL) salt

1. Combine all of the ingredients in a bowl and toss gently.

2. Stored in a sealed glass jar in the refrigerator, Salsa Fresca will keep for up to 2 days.

sun-dried tomato tapenade

Pictured on p. 135

This tapenade is brilliant in color and deep in flavor and contains far less oil than most other spreads. Try laying it with seasoned Nut Cheese (page 136) and serving it with crackers. It's also delightful thinned with water and served as a sauce over zucchini pasta (see pages 87 and 209).

½ cup (120 mL) sun-dried tomatoes, soaked in ¼ cup (60 mL) purified water for 3 hours and drained (reserve the soaking water)

½ Roma tomato, seeded and chopped

2 tablespoons (30 mL) pine nuts

1½ tablespoons (22 mL) chopped red onion

1 pitted date

1 clove garlic, crushed

2 fresh basil leaves, sliced into thin ribbons

¼ teaspoon (1 mL) salt

Pinch of dried oregano

1. Place all of the ingredients in a food processor fitted with the S blade and process just until combined; the mixture should be a little chunky. If necessary, add a few drops of the reserved sun-dried tomato soaking water to obtain the desired consistency.

2. Stored in an airtight container or a sealed glass jar in the refrigerator, Sun-Dried Tomato Tapenade will keep for up to 4 days.

note: A mini-processor works especially well for this recipe since it makes such a small quantity.

mexican corn and avocado salsa

YIELD: 3 CUPS/750 ML (3 SERVINGS)

Get in the mood for Mexican food. This mildly spicy salsa has a lively flavor and chunky texture. We enjoy it served with Red Hot Chips (page 129) and Salsa Fresca (page 139). It's also good wrapped in Fresh Corn Tortillas (page 126).

1½ cups (370 mL) cherry tomatoes, cut into quarters

1 ripe avocado, diced

1 cup (250 mL) fresh corn kernels

½ cup (120 mL) diced red bell pepper

½ cup (120 mL) chopped fresh cilantro, loosely packed

1 green onion, thinly sliced

1½ tablespoons (22 mL) freshly squeezed lime juice

1½ teaspoons (7 mL) flaxseed oil

1 clove garlic, crushed

½ teaspoon (2 mL) salt

¼ cup (60 mL) mung bean sprouts or Savory Seasoned Sunflower or Pumpkin Seeds (page 216)

1. Combine the tomatoes, avocado, corn, bell pepper, cilantro, green onion, lime juice, oil, garlic, and salt in a large bowl and toss gently.

2. Garnish with the bean sprouts and serve immediately.

NUTRITION NOTE This salsa provides over 100% of the RDA for vitamins A and C and is a rich source of omega-3 fatty acids.

sprouted chickpea hummus

YIELD: 1½ CUPS/370 ML (6 SERVINGS)

This hummus contains the flavors of the traditional version with a beautifully balanced combination of seasonings. While hummus is often served with flatbread, you can significantly reduce calories and boost nutrition by serving it on leaves of romaine lettuce topped with chopped tomatoes and sprouts.

HUMMUS

¾ cup (180 mL) sprouted chickpeas

¾ cup (180 mL) peeled and coarsely chopped zucchini

2½ tablespoons (37 mL) freshly squeezed lemon juice

2 cloves garlic, crushed

1 teaspoon (5 mL) ground coriander

1 teaspoon (5 mL) salt

½ teaspoon (2 mL) ground cumin

¼ teaspoon (1 mL) cayenne

6 tablespoons (90 mL) raw tahini

VEGETABLES FOR SERVING

1 head romaine lettuce

1 cup (250 mL) chopped ripe tomatoes

1 cup (250 mL) alfalfa sprouts

1. To make the hummus, combine the chickpea sprouts, zucchini, lemon juice, garlic, coriander, salt, cumin, and cayenne in a blender and process until smooth. Add a small amount of water, if needed, to facilitate processing and keep the mixture moving.

2. Add the tahini and process until completely smooth and creamy.

3. Serve on lettuce leaves with the tomatoes and sprouts.

4. Stored in a sealed glass jar in the refrigerator, Sprouted Chickpea Hummus will keep for up to 4 days.

NUTRITION NOTE One serving of Sprouted Chickpea Hummus provides about 150 calories, 6 grams of protein, and about 25% of the RDA for thiamin and iron.

sprouted lentil pâté with garlic and herbs

YIELD: 1½ CUPS/370 ML (4-6 SERVINGS)

U nlike most pâtés and dips, which are high in fat, this is a naturally low-fat yet flavorful pâté that is a fabulous snack or appetizer served with Flax Crackers (page 128) or Crudités (page 174). Alternatively, serve it alongside a salad to make a complete meal.

¾ cup (180 mL) sprouted lentils

3 tablespoons (45 mL) freshly squeezed lemon juice

3 tablespoons (45 mL) purified water

2 tablespoons (30 mL) Sun-Dried Tomato Powder (page 129)

2 tablespoons (30 mL) finely minced red onion

2 tablespoons (30 mL) minced fresh basil

2 tablespoons (30 mL) minced fresh parsley

1 tablespoon (15 mL) light miso

2 teaspoons (10 mL) nutritional yeast flakes

2 cloves garlic, crushed

½ teaspoon (2 mL) Italian seasoning

Pinch of salt

Pinch of freshly ground black pepper

1. Put the sprouted lentils in a food processor fitted with the S blade and process until smooth. Transfer to a medium bowl, add the remaining ingredients, and stir well.

2. Stored in an airtight container in the refrigerator, Sprouted Lentil Pâté with Garlic and Herbs will keep for up to 4 days.

NUTRITION NOTE Not only can lentils help lower cholesterol, they're of special benefit in managing blood sugar disorders since their high fiber content prevents blood sugar levels from rising rapidly after a meal. But this is not all lentils have to offer: they provide the greatest iron content of any legume. Of course, like most other legumes, they are also high in protein and very low in fat. This pâté has less than 100 calories per serving and is loaded with B vitamins, including over 25% of the RDA for vitamin B_{12} if made with Vegetarian Support Formula nutritional yeast.

broccoli pesto pâté

YIELD: 1½ CUPS/370 ML (3-4 SERVINGS)

Many of us love pesto, but often it's too rich for us to eat as much as we'd like. With this recipe, the fat has been reduced. Enjoy it as a spread on crackers, as a topping for salads, wrapped in romaine lettuce leaves, or as a dip with Crudités (page 174).

3 cups (750 mL) chopped broccoli florets

1½ cups (370 mL) fresh basil leaves, firmly packed

1 tablespoon (15 mL) flaxseed oil

2 teaspoons (10 mL) nutritional yeast flakes

1½ teaspoons (7 mL) light miso

1½ cloves garlic, crushed

¼ teaspoon (1 mL) salt

½ cup (120 mL) walnuts, soaked for 4 hours, rinsed, and drained

1. Put the broccoli into a large bowl and pour 1 quart (1 L) of nearly boiling water over it. Drain the broccoli after 1 minute and plunge it into cold water. This will turn the broccoli bright green and make it more palatable without negatively affecting the nutrients. Drain the broccoli well and place it on clean kitchen towels to remove any excess water. Set aside.

2. Combine the basil, oil, nutritional yeast flakes, miso, garlic, and salt in a food processor fitted with the S blade and pulse to chop the basil.

3. Add the walnuts and the reserved broccoli and process until the mixture is completely smooth and creamy.

4. Stored in a sealed glass jar in the refrigerator, Broccoli Pesto Pâté will keep for up to 3 days.

NUTRITION NOTE Broccoli makes a great addition to raw pâté, especially since it contains as much vitamin C as an orange, along with magnesium, the mineral that is central in green chlorophyll, and calcium. When you make pesto with Vegetarian Support Formula nutritional yeast, it's also a good source of B vitamins, including vitamin B_{12}.

broccoli-tahini pâté

If you enjoy the earthy flavor of broccoli and the creaminess of tahini, this will become a favorite in your house. It can be spread on crackers, used in nori wraps, or served as a dip with Crudités (page 174). For a tasty vegetable roll, wrap each serving of the pâté in a large collard or romaine lettuce leaf with chopped tomatoes, onions, and sprouts.

3 cups (750 mL) chopped broccoli florets

⅓ cup (80 mL) raw tahini

2 tablespoons (30 mL) sliced green onions

1 tablespoon (15 mL) ground flaxseeds

1 tablespoon (15 mL) nutritional yeast flakes

1 tablespoon (15 mL) tamari

1 tablespoon (15 mL) Dijon mustard or Hot Mustard (page 167)

2 large cloves garlic, crushed

Large pinch of cayenne

1. Put the broccoli into a large bowl and pour 1 quart (1 L) of nearly boiling water over it. Drain the broccoli after 1 minute and plunge it into cold water. This will turn the broccoli bright green and make it more palatable without negatively affecting the nutrients. Drain the broccoli well and place it on clean kitchen towels to remove any excess water.

2. Transfer the broccoli to a food processor fitted with the S blade. Add all of the remaining ingredients and process until the mixture is completely smooth and creamy.

3. Stored in a sealed glass jar in the refrigerator, Broccoli-Tahini Pâté will keep for up to 3 days.

NUTRITION NOTE This hearty pâté is high in protein (10 g per serving) and brings with it minerals (calcium, iron, magnesium, and zinc) and antioxidants (beta-carotene and vitamin C). A serving also provides your day's supply of riboflavin and thiamin, plus plenty of other B vitamins. Use Vegetarian Support Formula nutritional yeast, and you'll have a source of vitamin B_{12} too.

zucchini hummus

YIELD: 1⅔ CUPS/410 ML (5 SERVINGS)

This amazing, bean-free hummus is a big bonus for all of us who experience flatulence when we eat beans. It has all the flavor of traditional Middle Eastern hummus and is full of nutrients, including bone-strengthening calcium. Enjoy it served with Crudités (page 174) or in romaine lettuce boats with tomatoes and sprouts.

1 cup (250 mL) peeled and chopped zucchini, firmly packed

3½ tablespoons (52 mL) freshly squeezed lemon juice

1 tablespoon (15 mL) flaxseed oil

4 cloves garlic

1 teaspoon (5 mL) paprika

1 teaspoon (5 mL) salt

¼ teaspoon (1 mL) ground cumin (optional)

Pinch of cayenne

½ cup (120 mL) raw tahini

⅓ cup (80 mL) sesame seeds, soaked for 4 hours, rinsed, and drained

1. Combine the zucchini, lemon juice, oil, garlic, paprika, salt, optional cumin, and cayenne in a blender and process until smooth.

2. Add the tahini and sesame seeds and process until completely smooth and creamy.

3. Stored in a sealed glass jar in the refrigerator, Zucchini Hummus will keep for up to 4 days.

note: This recipe is best made in a high-speed blender. However, it can be made successfully in a standard blender if it is processed in two batches. Alternatively, it can be made in a food processor, although the result will be a little different. A food processor will not pulverize the sesame seeds, so the mixture will have whole sesame seeds in it rather than being smooth and creamy.

not tuna salad

YIELD: 1½ CUPS/370 ML (6 SERVINGS)

Fresh and full of the flavor of the sea, this salad can be enjoyed with crackers or Crudités (page 174) or spread inside a nori roll. Other popular ways to serve it are as the central attraction on a composed salad or stuffed into a ripe, juicy tomato, red bell pepper, or hollowed cucumber. Alternatively, roll it in romaine lettuce or collard leaves, Fresh Corn Tortillas (page 126), or other wraps, or spread it between slices of Sprouted Grain Bread (page 122) with tomatoes, raw vegan mayonnaise, and lettuce. Any way you can imagine eating tuna salad, you can enjoy Not Tuna Salad.

1½ cups (370 mL) almonds, soaked for 24 hours, rinsed, and drained

1 cup (250 mL) sunflower seeds, soaked for 4–6 hours, rinsed, and drained

½ cup (120 mL) purified water, as needed

½ cup (120 mL) minced celery

½ cup (120 mL) minced red onion

½ cup (120 mL) minced fresh parsley

⅓ cup (80 mL) freshly squeezed lemon juice

1 tablespoon (15 mL) kelp powder

1½ teaspoons (7 mL) fresh dill weed, or 1 teaspoon (5 mL) dried

½ teaspoon (2 mL) salt

1. Process the almonds and sunflower seeds through a Champion or Green Life Juicer fitted with the homogenizing plate. If necessary, use very a small amount of the water, alternating it with the nuts and seeds, to facilitate processing. Alternatively, process the almonds and sunflower seeds in a food processor fitted with the S blade, although the texture will not be as fine.

2. Transfer the mixture to a large bowl and stir in the remaining ingredients.

3. Stored in an airtight container in the refrigerator, Not Tuna Salad will keep for up to 1 week.

variations

NOT SALMON SALAD: Add ½ cup (120 mL) carrot pulp (from making carrot juice) for color, and season the mixture with fresh or dried dill weed to taste.

NOT TUNA CRACKERS: Put ¾ cup (180 mL) Not Tuna Salad on top of a nori sheet, and evenly spread a thin (⅛-inch/3-mm) layer right to the edges. Place another nori sheet on top, press it into place, and slice evenly into 12 squares. Dehydrate at 105 degrees F/40 degrees C for about 24 hours, or until crisp.

NUTRITION NOTE This dish provides an impressive 13 grams of protein and 6 grams of fiber per serving. It also packs over 35% of the RDA for biotin, riboflavin, thiamin, and vitamins E and K.

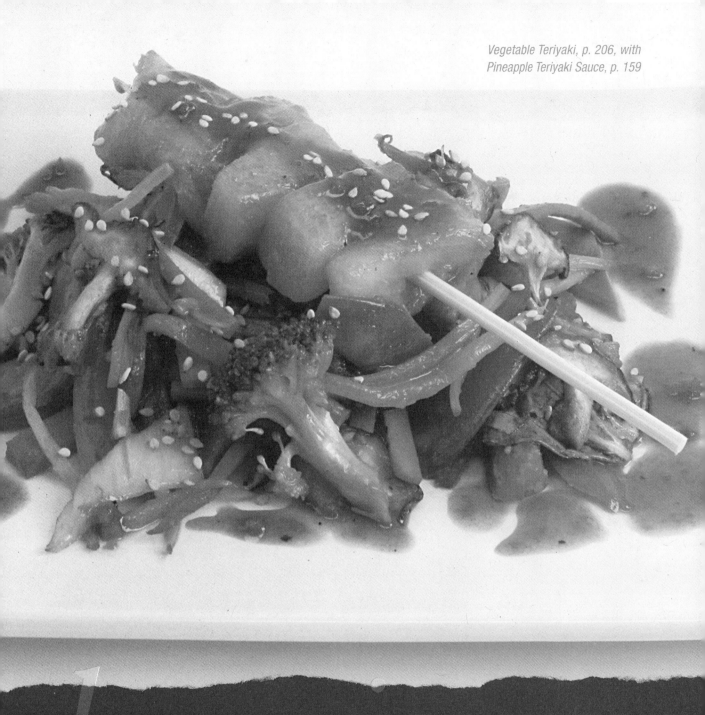

Vegetable Teriyaki, p. 206, with Pineapple Teriyaki Sauce, p. 159

DRESSINGS, MARINADES, AND SAUCES

sweet dijon dressing

YIELD: 1¼ CUPS/310 ML (6 SERVINGS)

This is one of the favorite dressings served at the Living Light Café and Cuisine To Go. It goes great with any salad, especially apple salads. It can also be used as a vegetable marinade. Dijon mustard is known for its bright, sharp flavor, in varieties ranging from mild to hot.

1 cup (250 mL) peeled and chopped zucchini

¼ cup (60 mL) freshly squeezed lemon juice

2 tablespoons (30 mL) flaxseed oil

1½ tablespoons (22 mL) minced red onion

1½ tablespoons (22 mL) agave syrup

1 tablespoon (15 mL) Dijon mustard or Hot Mustard (page 167)

1 tablespoon (15 mL) ground flaxseeds

1 teaspoon (5 mL) dark miso

½ teaspoon (2 mL) salt

1 clove garlic, crushed

Pinch of freshly ground black pepper

1. Combine all of the ingredients in a blender and process until smooth.

2. Stored in a sealed glass jar in the refrigerator, Sweet Dijon Dressing will keep for up to 4 days.

note: If you choose to use Hot Mustard rather than Dijon, you may want to use a little less, as it will definitely add some heat.

NUTRITION NOTE This dressing covers your requirements for omega-3 fatty acids with almost 3 grams per serving.

creamy hemp dressing

Salad dressings often serve only to smother a beautiful salad—particularly the bottled oil-and-vinegar or water-and-sugar concoctions found on grocery store shelves. This delicious, creamy dressing is a good example of what a great salad dressing can be. Hempseeds are a fun and interesting addition, contributing a slightly sweet, nutty flavor to the dressing. Enjoy Creamy Hemp Dressing over salads and slaws, or as a flavorful base for creamy soups.

½ cup (120 mL) freshly squeezed lemon juice

½ cup (120 mL) coarsely chopped celery

¼ cup (60 mL) flaxseed oil

¼ cup (60 mL) hempseeds

¼ cup (60 mL) nutritional yeast flakes

¼ cup (60 mL) purified water

2 tablespoons (30 mL) chopped fresh basil or dill weed, or 2 teaspoons (10 mL) dried

2 tablespoons (30 mL) coarsely chopped onion

4 teaspoons (20 mL) light miso

2 teaspoons (10 mL) agave syrup

2 teaspoons (10 mL) tamari

1. Combine all of the ingredients in a blender and process until smooth.

2. Stored in a sealed glass jar in the refrigerator, Creamy Hemp Dressing will keep for up to 2 weeks.

NUTRITION NOTE Creamy Hemp Dressing has amazing flavor and an outstanding nutrition profile. One serving provides over 50% of the RDA for four B vitamins and over 40% of the RDA for vitamin B_{12}. The hempseeds provide a highly impressive combination of nutrients, including high-quality protein, minerals, vitamins, and a fine balance of essential fatty acids.

italian herb dressing

YIELD: 1⅛ CUPS/280 ML (6 SERVINGS)

Spice up your salad with this light dressing featuring the flavors of Italy. Most Italian dressings contain vinegar, which causes digestive problems and bloating for many people. This quick and simple dressing calls for lemon juice instead of vinegar and is just as delicious, plus it's a good source of omega-3 fatty acids due to the flaxseed oil. It also makes a great marinade to soften vegetables.

1 cup (250 mL) peeled and chopped zucchini

¼ cup (60 mL) freshly squeezed lemon juice

2 tablespoons (30 mL) flaxseed oil

2 tablespoons (30 mL) agave syrup

1¼ teaspoons (6 mL) Italian seasoning

1 teaspoon (5 mL) onion powder

1 teaspoon (5 mL) ground flaxseeds

¾ teaspoon (4 mL) salt

1 clove garlic, crushed

Pinch of powdered mustard

1. Combine all of the ingredients in a blender and process until smooth. Alternatively, combine the ingredients in a bowl and whisk to blend.

2. Stored in a sealed glass jar in the refrigerator, Italian Herb Dressing will keep for up to 4 days.

liquid gold dressing

YIELD: 1 CUP/250 ML (4 SERVINGS)

This delicious dressing is adapted from the nutrition books *The New Becoming Vegetarian*, *Becoming Vegan*, and *Raising Vegetarian Children*. Zucchini and ground flaxseeds were added to reduce the amount of oil needed and to create a thick, rich consistency and increase the omega-3 fatty acid content. But the flavor of the dressing is what will make you want to have it again and again!

1 cup (250 mL) peeled and chopped zucchini

¼ cup (60 mL) freshly squeezed lemon juice

¼ cup (60 mL) nutritional yeast flakes

2 tablespoons (30 mL) flaxseed oil

2 tablespoons (30 mL) tamari

2 teaspoons (10 mL) ground flaxseeds

1 teaspoon (5 mL) Dijon mustard

1 teaspoon (5 mL) agave syrup

½ teaspoon (2 mL) ground cumin

½ teaspoon (2 mL) crushed garlic (optional)

1. Combine all of the ingredients in a blender and process until smooth.

2. Stored in a sealed glass jar in the refrigerator, Liquid Gold Dressing will keep for up to 2 weeks.

variation

GREEN GODDESS DRESSING: Omit the Dijon mustard and cumin and add 1 cup (250 mL) of chopped fresh herbs (basil, oregano, and/or parsley work very well) and increase the garlic to 1 teaspoon (5 mL).

NUTRITION NOTE One serving (¼ cup/60 mL) of Liquid Gold Dressing provides your day's supply of omega-3 fatty acids and is packed with riboflavin and other B vitamins (folate, niacin, thiamin, and vitamin B_6). When it's made with Red Star Vegetarian Support Formula nutritional yeast, it also delivers 40% of your vitamin B_{12} for the day!

pineapple lemongrette

I f you find salad dressing a little humdrum, this fantastic fusion of sweet-and-tangy flavors is guaranteed to tingle your taste buds. Serve it over fruit or vegetable salads. It's especially good on bitter or spicy greens.

½ cup (120 mL) peeled and chopped zucchini

4 ounces (114 g) unsweetened dried pineapple, soaked in ½ cup (120 mL) purified water for 1 hour and drained (see note)

2 tablespoons (30 mL) flaxseed oil

1–2 tablespoons (15–30 mL) purified water, as needed

1 tablespoon (15 mL) freshly squeezed lemon juice

1 teaspoon (5 mL) Hot Mustard (page 167) or Dijon mustard

½ teaspoon (2 mL) salt

1 clove garlic, crushed

¼ teaspoon (1 mL) freshly ground black pepper

1. Combine all of the ingredients in a blender and process until smooth.

2. Stored in a sealed glass jar in the refrigerator, Pineapple Lemongrette will keep for up to 4 days.

note: If dried pineapple isn't available, substitute ½ cup (120 mL) fresh pineapple and add ½–1 teaspoon (2–5 mL) of agave syrup for additional sweetness, if needed.

NUTRITION NOTE Besides being delicious, pineapple contains enzymes that may aid your digestion. And one serving of Pineapple Lemongrette provides fewer than 80 calories!

savory seed dressing

This nourishing dressing is easy to make and can transform an ordinary salad into a full meal. The nutty taste can be varied using different seeds and a variety of herbs and seasonings depending on your mood.

½ cup (120 mL) pumpkin, sesame, or sunflower seeds

1 cup (250 mL) purified water

2 cloves garlic

¼ cup (60 mL) freshly squeezed lemon juice

¼ cup (60 mL) freshly squeezed orange juice

3 tablespoons (45 mL) tamari or light miso

3 tablespoons (45 mL) ground flaxseeds

2 tablespoons (30 mL) flaxseed oil (optional)

1 teaspoon (5 mL) powdered mustard

½ teaspoon (2 mL) dried basil

½ teaspoon (2 mL) dried oregano

½ teaspoon (2 mL) dried thyme

1. Combine the seeds, water, and garlic in a blender and process until smooth and creamy. Add a little more water to facilitate processing, if necessary.

2. Add the lemon juice, orange juice, tamari, flaxseeds, optional oil, powdered mustard, basil, oregano, and thyme and process again until well combined. Add a little more water if the dressing is too thick.

3. Stored in a sealed glass jar in the refrigerator, Savory Seed Dressing will keep for up to 4 days.

NUTRITION NOTE Savory Seed Dressing is rich in vitamin E and omega-3 fatty acids. Seeds also are good sources of a variety of minerals.

tahini-ginger dressing

YIELD: 1½ CUPS/370 ML (6-8 SERVINGS)

Creamy, sweet, pungent, and perfectly balanced in flavor, this outstanding dressing is one of our favorites on broccoli, cabbage, greens, or any kind of vegetable salad. The combination of sesame, ginger, and garlic gives it a snappy taste that can also be enjoyed as an Asian-style noodle sauce or as a dip by simply reducing the amount of water.

1 cup (250 mL) purified water

2 tablespoons (30 mL) freshly squeezed lemon juice

2 tablespoons (30 mL) tamari

1 tablespoon (15 mL) agave syrup

2 teaspoons (10 mL) grated fresh ginger

2 cloves garlic, crushed

½ cup (120 mL) raw tahini

1. Combine all of the ingredients in a blender, adding the water first and tahini last, and process until smooth.

2. Stored in a sealed glass jar in the refrigerator, Tahini-Ginger Dressing will keep for up to 1 week.

tomato-basil dressing

YIELD: 1¾ CUPS/430 ML (8 SERVINGS)

This easy-to-make dressing is a popular standard at the Living Light Café and Cuisine To Go, served over a fresh garden salad topped with sliced avocado and seasoned seeds. Accompanied by a side of Pizza Flax Crackers (page 129), it makes a complete and satisfying meal.

2½ ripe tomatoes, seeded and coarsely chopped

3 tablespoons (45 mL) chopped fresh basil leaves

2 tablespoons (30 mL) freshly squeezed lemon juice

1½ tablespoons (22 mL) flaxseed oil

1 tablespoon (15 mL) Sun-Dried Tomato Powder (see page 129)

1 tablespoon (15 mL) agave syrup (optional)

1 clove garlic, crushed

½ teaspoon (2 mL) salt

¼ teaspoon (1 mL) Italian seasoning

Pinch of powdered mustard

Pinch of freshly ground black pepper

1. Combine all of the ingredients in a blender and process until smooth.

2. Stored in a sealed glass jar in the refrigerator, Tomato-Basil Dressing will keep for up to 2 days.

note: If tomatoes are out of season, a little agave syrup or additional sun-dried tomato powder will intensify the flavor and make the dressing sweeter.

NUTRITION NOTE Tomato-Basil Dressing a good source of vitamin E and omega-3 fatty acids.

fat-free tomato-herb dressing

Keep a lid on calories, not on flavor, with this easy-to-make, fat-free dressing. Even after you've achieved your weight-loss goals, you'll consider this a keeper.

1½ cups (370 mL) coarsely chopped ripe tomatoes

1 cup (250 mL) peeled and chopped zucchini

¼ cup (60 mL) chopped celery

2 tablespoons (30 mL) freshly squeezed lemon juice

1 tablespoon (15 mL) agave syrup (optional)

2 teaspoons (10 mL) Italian seasoning

2 cloves garlic

1 teaspoon (5 mL) onion powder

½ teaspoon (2 mL) chopped red onion

½ teaspoon (2 mL) salt

Pinch of freshly ground black pepper

1. Combine all of the ingredients in a blender and process until smooth.

2. Stored in a sealed glass jar in the refrigerator, Fat-Free Tomato-Herb Dressing will keep for up to 2 days.

note: If tomatoes are out of season, a little agave syrup will intensify the flavor and make the dressing sweeter.

NUTRITION NOTE With only 40 calories per serving, this dressing provides over 20% of the RDA for chromium and vitamin C, and it has a good supply of carotenoids.

bon bon sauce

This Asian-style sesame sauce can be used on just about anything. If you thin it with water, it's a tasty salad dressing; if you use less water, it's a great vegetable dip, spread, or filling for celery sticks. Enjoy it as a dipping sauce for Vegetable Sushimaki with Spicy Miso Paste (page 204) or Vietnamese Salad Rolls (page 205), or use it instead of mayonnaise for cabbage slaw. However you serve it, Bon Bon Sauce is a guaranteed crowd pleaser.

½ cup (120 mL) raw tahini

2 tablespoons (30 mL) grated fresh ginger

2 tablespoons (30 mL) freshly squeezed lemon juice

2 tablespoons (30 mL) agave syrup

2 tablespoons (30 mL) tamari

1 clove garlic, crushed

1. Combine of the ingredients in a blender and process until smooth. Add a small amount of purified water as needed to form a thick sauce.

2. Stored in a sealed glass jar in the refrigerator, Bon Bon Sauce will keep for up to 1 week.

cashew-dill sauce

cashew

Cashews provide the perfect base for thick, creamy sauces. The addition of pine nuts makes the sauce taste less like cashew cream and more like real cream. The less water you add, the thicker the cream will be. Use this luscious sauce over delicately flavored vegetables like cucumbers and zucchini, or add it to soups and dressings to make them creamier.

½ cup (120 mL) cashews

½ cup (120 mL) pine nuts

⅓ cup (80 mL) freshly squeezed lemon juice

2 tablespoons (30 mL) agave syrup

1½ tablespoons (22 mL) minced fresh dill weed

1 tablespoon (15 mL) onion powder

1 teaspoon (5 mL) salt

1. Combine the cashews, pine nuts, lemon juice, agave syrup, half of the dill weed, the onion powder, and salt in a blender and process until smooth and creamy. Add purified water as needed to make a thick sauce. Stir in the remaining dill weed.

2. Stored in a sealed glass jar, Cashew-Dill Sauce will keep for up to 1 week in the refrigerator or up to 3 months in the freezer.

variations

■ Replace the dill weed other fresh herbs, such as basil, cilantro, sage, or savory.

■ Add fresh garlic to taste.

NUTRITION NOTE A single serving of Cashew-Dill Sauce provides a host of minerals—over 15% of the RDA for copper, magnesium, manganese, phosphorus, and zinc.

pineapple teriyaki sauce

YIELD: 1¼ CUPS/310 ML (5 SERVINGS)

The flavor dynamic of teriyaki sauce is what makes it one of the most popular sauces in the world. It's sweet, pungent, salty, and explosive in flavor, making it a versatile sauce to have on hand. The brilliance of pineapple adds even more irresistible aroma and flavor to this enticing sauce. Use Pineapple Teriyaki Sauce to marinate vegetables, or try it as a glaze on vegetable or tropical fruit kabobs. It can also be used to flavor salad dressings or season Wild Rice Pilaf (page 200). It also makes a great dip for Vegetable Sushimaki with Spicy Miso Paste (page 204). For a unique and delicious version of teriyaki almonds, toss the sauce with almonds that have been soaked and then dehydrated until crispy.

½ cup (120 mL) cubed pineapple

¼ cup (60 mL) raw sesame oil

¼ cup (60 mL) sliced red onion

3 tablespoons (45 mL) tamari

2 tablespoons (30 mL) evaporated cane juice

2 cloves garlic

1½ teaspoons (7 mL) freshly squeezed lemon juice

1 teaspoon (5 mL) grated fresh ginger

Pinch of freshly ground black pepper

Pinch of cayenne

1. Combine all of the ingredients in a blender and process until smooth.

2. Transfer to a 1-quart (1-L) glass jar and dehydrate uncovered at 115 degrees F/45 degrees C for at least 2 hours, or until thick. Alternatively, serve the sauce immediately (it will be thinner if it is not dehydrated).

3. Stored in a sealed glass jar in the refrigerator, Pineapple Teriyaki Sauce will keep for up to 1 week.

spicy sweet-and-sour sauce

spicy

This sauce is a piquant combination of sweet-and-tangy flavors with a spicy kick from jalapeño chiles. It's a lovely accompaniment to any meal with an Asian flair. Serve it as a dipping sauce with Vegetable Sushimaki with Spicy Miso Paste (page 204) or Vietnamese Salad Rolls (page 205), or use it as a sauce for Asian-style vegetable dishes.

1 cup (250 mL) diced ripe mango

1 lemon, juiced

3 tablespoons (45 mL) evaporated cane juice

3 tablespoons (45 mL) agave syrup

2 tablespoons (30 mL) minced red onion

2 red jalapeño chiles, seeded and minced

1 teaspoon (5 mL) grated fresh ginger

1 clove garlic, crushed

¼ teaspoon (1 mL) Hot Lava Sauce (page 171; optional)

¼ teaspoon (1 mL) salt

1. Combine all of the ingredients in a blender and process until smooth.

2. Adjust the flavors to suit your taste by adding more agave syrup, lemon juice, Hot Lava Sauce, or salt, if desired.

3. Stored in a sealed glass jar in the refrigerator, Spicy Sweet-and-Sour Sauce will keep for up to 3 days.

NUTRITION NOTE With less than 75 calories per serving, this sauce has nearly 20% of the RDA for vitamin C.

pizza sauce

This thick, rich pizza sauce mimics the real thing and tastes like it was cooked for hours. It's easy to make and has the fresh flavor of fennel, which is what sets it apart from marinara sauce and makes it a perfect topping for raw pizza crust, like our Sprouted Seed Pizza Crusts (page 132). Or try layering it with Nut Cheese (page 136) and using it as a dip.

1½ cups (370 mL) Roma tomatoes, seeded, drained, and chopped

¼ cup (60 mL) Sun-Dried Tomato Powder (see page 129)

1 tablespoon (15 mL) extra-virgin olive oil

3 fresh basil leaves, minced

1 clove garlic, crushed

1½ teaspoons (7 mL) minced onion

¾ teaspoon (4 mL) minced fresh oregano

½ teaspoon (2 mL) salt

½ teaspoon (2 mL) freshly squeezed lemon juice

½ teaspoon (2 mL) agave syrup

¼ teaspoon (1 mL) ground fennel

Pinch of freshly ground black pepper

1. Combine all of the ingredients in a blender and process until smooth.
2. Store in a sealed glass jar in the refrigerator, Pizza Sauce will keep for up to 2 days.

note: If the juice from the tomatoes is not completely drained, the mixture will separate slightly and the liquid from the tomatoes will rise to the top. However, the sauce will thicken as the Sun-Dried Tomato Powder absorbs the liquid. If the sauce is still too thin for your liking, drain off a little of the juice or add a little more Sun-Dried Tomato Powder. Adjust the seasonings as necessary.

NUTRITION NOTE With about 100 calories per serving, Pizza Sauce is a nutritional bargain, providing over 10% of the RDA for seven vitamins and eight minerals, and a host of protective phytochemicals.

pesto sauce

Quick and easy to prepare, pesto is a favorite over raw vegetable pasta (see page 87) and pizza. It can also be used in salad dressings and to flavor soups. With its distinctive flavor, basil is the most popular herb used to prepare pesto, but pesto can be made with other herbs, alone or in combination, such as cilantro, mint, or parsley.

1 cup (250 mL) chopped zucchini

2 cups (500 mL) fresh basil leaves, firmly packed

2 tablespoons (30 mL) flaxseed oil

1 tablespoon (15 mL) light miso

1 tablespoon (15 mL) nutritional yeast flakes

2 cloves garlic, crushed

¼ teaspoon (1 mL) salt

½ cup (120 mL) walnuts

1. Place the zucchini in a food processor fitted with the S blade and process until smooth.

2. Add the basil, oil, miso, nutritional yeast flakes, garlic, and salt and pulse a few times to coarsely chop the basil.

3. Add the walnuts and process until the desired consistency is achieved. Do not overprocess the mixture or the oil from the walnuts will separate and the mixture will become too oily. The texture should be creamy, with tiny specks of walnuts throughout.

4. Stored in a sealed glass jar in the refrigerator, Pesto Sauce will keep for up to 4 days. Alternatively, freeze Pesto Sauce in ice cube trays and then transfer the frozen cubes to an airtight container. Stored in the freezer, Pesto Sauce will keep for up to 3 months.

NUTRITION NOTE This version of pesto provides an impressive host of vitamins and minerals, along with a near-perfect balance of omega-3 to omega-6 fatty acids.

marinara sauce

This marinara is a quick, low-fat sauce with less than 50 calories per serving. People often comment on its lively fresh taste compared to cooked sauce. Fresh marinara is great over spiralized zucchini "pasta" (see page 87) or as a pizza topping, but it also makes a great dip for Crudités (page 174). If there is any left over, add it to soups or salad dressings. You can even use this versatile sauce as a base for Flax Crackers (page 128) or Fresh Corn Tortillas (page 126).

2 Roma tomatoes, seeded and chopped

3 tablespoons (45 mL) Sun-Dried Tomato Powder (see page 129)

1 tablespoon (15 mL) finely minced onion

1 tablespoon (15 mL) minced fresh basil leaves

1 tablespoon (15 mL) minced fresh oregano

1 clove garlic, crushed

¼ teaspoon (1 mL) salt

Pinch of freshly ground black pepper

1. Place the tomatoes in a colander and allow any liquid to drain. (Drink the wonderful juice or add it to another recipe.) When the tomatoes are thoroughly drained, transfer them to a food processor fitted with the S blade and process briefly, just until slightly chunky.

2. Add the Sun-Dried Tomato Powder, onion, basil, oregano, garlic, salt, and pepper and pulse to combine.

3. Let the sauce sit for 10 minutes before serving to allow it to thicken. If it's still too thin, drain off a little of the liquid.

4. Stored in a tightly sealed glass jar in the refrigerator, Marinara Sauce will keep for up to 3 days.

variations

RED BELL PEPPER MARINARA: Add ¼ red bell pepper, chopped, along with the tomatoes.

RICH MARINARA: Add 1 tablespoon (15 mL) of extra-virgin olive oil.

SPICY MARINARA: Add a pinch of cayenne.

NUTRITION NOTE Thanks to fresh, ripe tomatoes, Marinara Sauce provides a nice mix of antioxidants, including lycopene and other carotenoids, as well as vitamin C.

onion-shiitake gravy

YIELD: 1½ CUPS/370 ML (8 SERVINGS)

Tahini forms the creamy, calcium-rich base of this gravy. Serve it with Zoom Burgers (page 208). It's also great over spiralized zucchini pasta (see page 87) or as an alternative to marinara sauce. This gravy is rich and satisfying no matter how you serve it.

1¼ cups (310 mL) warm purified water, more or less as needed

⅓ cup (80 mL) raw tahini

⅓ cup (80 mL) Dried Shiitake Mushroom Powder (see sidebar)

1½ tablespoons (22 mL) tamari

4 teaspoons (20 mL) onion powder

1 teaspoon (5 mL) agave syrup

1. Combine all of the ingredients in a blender and process until smooth and creamy, using only as much water as needed to facilitate processing and achieve the desired consistency.

2. Stored in a sealed glass jar, Onion-Shiitake Gravy will keep for up to 4 days in the refrigerator or up to 3 months in the freezer.

Dried Shiitake Mushroom Powder

To make Dried Shiitake Mushroom Powder, place 2½ ounces (70 g) dried shiitake mushrooms in a high-powered blender and grind them into a fine powder. Stored in a glass jar in the pantry, Dried Shiitake Mushroom Powder will keep for at least 1 month.

Zoom Burgers, p. 208, and Crispy Sweet Onion Rings, p. 134,
with Cashew Mayonnaise, p. 166, Hot Mustard, p. 167,
and Real Tomato Ketchup, p. 168

condiments

CONDIMENTS AND CHUTNEYS

cashew mayonnaise

YIELD: 1-1¼ CUPS/250-310 ML (16 SERVINGS)

Even most health-conscious eaters want to enjoy a luscious spread similar to their favorite mayonnaise. This one is made from cashews and is easy to prepare using a blender. Add it to dressings, dips, and sandwiches.

1 cup (250 ml) cashews, soaked for 2 hours, rinsed, and drained

¼ cup (60 ml) purified water

¼ cup (60 ml) freshly squeezed lemon juice

2 pitted soft dates

1 teaspoon (5 ml) salt

1 teaspoon (5 ml) onion powder

½ teaspoon (2 ml) garlic powder

Pinch of freshly ground white pepper

2 tablespoons (30 ml) extra-virgin olive oil

2 tablespoons (30 ml) flaxseed oil

1. Combine the cashews, water, lemon juice, dates, salt, onion powder, garlic powder, and pepper in a blender and process until smooth.

2. With the blender running, add the olive oil and flaxseed oil in a steady stream until they are emulsified.

3. Stored in a tightly sealed glass jar in the refrigerator, Cashew Mayonnaise will keep for up to 4 weeks.

NUTRITION NOTE This mayo is a good source of magnesium and zinc (because of the cashews) and omega-3 fatty acids (due to the flaxseed oil).

hot mustard

Hot, zesty, and pungent, mustard has long been a culinary favorite in American and European cultures. There are three types of mustard seeds: white (or yellow), brown (or Asian), and black. White mustard seeds are larger than brown but a bit less pungent. You can blend the two to make what is known as English mustard. Mustard seeds can be stored for up to a year in a dry, dark place. Prepared mustard becomes milder with age, so if it's too hot at first, keep it in the refrigerator for a few weeks and it will mellow.

9 pitted dates

¾ cup (180 mL) mustard seeds, soaked for 8–12 hours, rinsed, and drained

½ cup (120 mL) freshly squeezed lemon juice

2 tablespoons (30 mL) tamari

1. If the dates are very hard and dry, soak them in warm purified water for a few minutes to soften. Drain before using.

2. Combine all of the ingredients in a blender and process into a smooth paste.

3. Stored in a sealed glass jar in the refrigerator, Hot Mustard will keep for up to 2 months.

note: If you prefer a sweeter mustard, add 1 or 2 more dates to taste.

real tomato ketchup

YIELD: 2 CUPS/500 ML (12 SERVINGS)

This is called "real" tomato ketchup because it is exactly how tomato ketchup should taste—fresh and full of vitality! The secret ingredient in this lively condiment is the tamarind fruit; it's both tart and sweet. Purchase tamarind in the pod (or removed from the pod and pressed into bars) at Asian, Indian, or Latin American markets. Tamarind can be used in sauces and dressings to enliven the flavor and reduce the need for salt.

2 cups (500 mL) chopped ripe tomatoes

6 tablespoons (90 mL) Sun-Dried Tomato Powder (see page 129)

1½ tablespoons (22 mL) evaporated cane juice

1 tablespoon (15 mL) freshly squeezed lemon juice

1 tablespoon (15 mL) tamarind paste, or 2 teaspoons (10 mL) additional lemon juice

¾ teaspoon (4 mL) salt

Pinch of freshly ground white pepper

1. Combine all of the ingredients in a blender or a food processor fitted with the S blade and process until smooth.

2. Stored in a sealed glass jar in the refrigerator, Real Tomato Ketchup will keep for up to 1 week.

berry-date jam

YIELD: 2 CUPS/500 ML (6-8 SERVINGS)

Are you surprised to find a recipe for jam in a book about weight loss? While commercial jam is essentially fruit-flavored sugar, this jam actually contributes to your nutrient intake. You'll love the simplicity of this recipe, which is sweetened only with fruit and contains no processed sugar. Enjoy a hearty serving of this jam with Date and Walnut Scones (page 124) or Sprouted Multi-Grain Bread (page 123).

2 cups (500 mL) fresh berries

1½ cups (370 mL) pitted dates, packed

1. Place the berries in a blender and process until smooth.

2. Loosely separate the dates and add them to the blender. Process until smooth. If the dates are very dry, blend for 1 minute, then turn the blender off and allow the dates to soak in the puréed berries for a few minutes to soften. Then continue blending until smooth.

3. Stored in a sealed glass jar, Berry-Date Jam will keep for up to 2 days in the refrigerator or up to 4 months in the freezer.

variations: Other sweet dried fruits can be used in place of the dates to thicken and intensify the sweetness of this jam. Try dried cherries, figs, pineapple, raisins, or even prunes.

note: If fresh berries are not available, an equal amount of frozen berries may be used. Defrost them and allow them to come to room temperature before blending.

cabbage kraut

Fermented foods, including cabbage kraut, have been used for centuries and touted as health promoters for the beneficial bacteria they provide to keep our intestinal tracts healthy and in good working order.

1 cabbage, very finely shredded (10 cups/2.5 L; reserve several cabbage leaves to cover the kraut)

1 teaspoon (5 mL) salt

1. Put the cabbage into a large bowl. Add the salt and gently massage it into the cabbage until liquid starts to release.

2. Let the cabbage rest for 10 minutes and massage it again. Repeat as often as necessary until the cabbage is very juicy.

3. Pack the mixture firmly into a large jar, crock, or bowl. Press the cabbage down until the liquid rises above it about ⅛ inch (3 mm).

4. If you are using a large jar for your kraut, put a weight on top of the cabbage, such as a small jar filled with water. If you're using a crock or bowl, put a plate on top of the cabbage and then a weight. Cover everything with a clean dish towel.

5. Allow the kraut to ferment in a cool, dark place for 3–14 days, depending on the degree of sourness you desire.

6. Once the kraut is ready, store it in sealed glass jars in the refrigerator. Cabbage Kraut will keep for up to several months.

variations

- If you wish to reduce the salt, run half of the cabbage through a Champion or Green Star Juicer fitted with the homogenizing plate, and add both the juice and the pulp to the shredded cabbage. This will add more liquid to the kraut.

- Add small amounts of other root or cruciferous vegetables, such as carrot, beet, or broccoli.

- Add seasonings and herbs to taste, such as caraway seeds, fresh dill weed, freshly squeezed lemon juice, or garlic.

NUTRITION NOTE Fresh cabbage kraut, used in judicious amounts, is a cornerstone of many "living food" diets. It's particularly good for people who have undergone any kind of antibiotic treatment. You may find it best to begin with 2 tablespoons (30 mL) and build up to ¼ cup (60 mL) per serving.

hot lava sauce

This brilliant red sauce adds heat and tang to any savory dish. Ripe bell peppers are the Christmas ornaments of the vegetable world, with beautifully shaped, glossy exteriors that come in a wide array of vivid colors ranging from red, yellow, and orange to purple, brown, and even black. Green bell peppers are unripe fruit, which is why they cause digestive difficulties for many people. Make sure to choose plump, vibrantly red peppers for this pungent and spicy sauce. For a less spicy sauce, use less habanero chile.

1 red bell pepper, coarsely chopped

¼ cup (60 mL) coarsely chopped red onion

1½ tablespoons (22 mL) freshly squeezed lemon juice

1 tablespoon (15 mL) paprika

1 habanero chile, with seeds, coarsely chopped

1 teaspoon (5 mL) evaporated cane juice

½ teaspoon (2 mL) salt

1 clove garlic

1. Combine all of the ingredients in a blender and process until smooth.

2. Stored in a sealed glass jar in the refrigerator, Hot Lava Sauce will keep for up to 6 days (if Hot Lava Sauce is kept at room temperature, it will spoil much more quickly).

red pepper rémoulade

YIELD: 1½ CUPS/370 ML (6 SERVINGS)

Rémoulade is a thick, slightly sweet French sauce similar to thin mayonnaise. This version showcases the lively red color of ripe bell peppers and serves as a wonderful complement to vegetables, croquettes, crêpes, and burgers.

1½ cups (370 mL) chopped red bell peppers

½ cup (120 mL) pine nuts or cashews, soaked, rinsed, and drained

¼ cup (60 mL) purified water

1½ tablespoons (20 mL) chopped fresh parsley

1½ teaspoons (7 mL) paprika

1½ teaspoons (7 mL) Hot Mustard (page 167)

1 clove garlic, crushed

¼ teaspoon (1 mL) salt

¼ teaspoon (1 mL) freshly ground black pepper

1½ teaspoons (7 mL) agave syrup (optional)

1. Combine the bell peppers, pine nuts, water, parsley, paprika, Hot Mustard, garlic, salt, and pepper in a blender and process until smooth. Taste and sweeten with the optional agave syrup, if needed.

2. Stored in a sealed glass jar in the refrigerator, Red Pepper Rémoulade will keep for up to 2 days.

variation: Thin the rémoulade with water and used it as a dressing for fruit or vegetable salads.

note: The sweetness of this rémoulade is affected by the natural flavor of the bell peppers, so if the peppers are not sweet, agave syrup can be added to achieve the desired flavor. Agave syrup may also be added if the mustard is freshly made and/or very hot, since the syrup will mellow its heat.

NUTRITION NOTE With this rémoulade you can enjoy the nutritional perks of red bell peppers, which are overflowing with carotenoids and vitamins C and K. Of course, the nuts further boost the mineral content of this sauce.

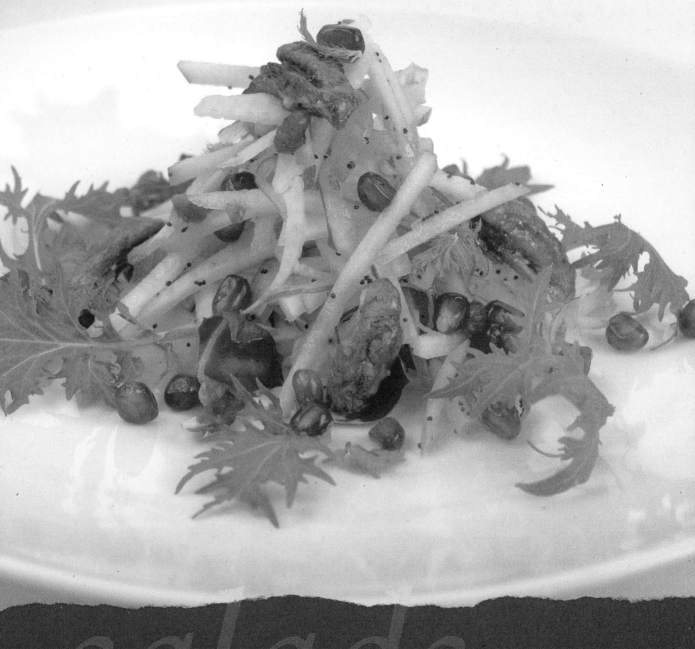

Apples and Walnuts on Baby Greens with
Poppy Seed Dressing, p. 179

salads

SALADS

crudités

Crudités, or raw vegetable sticks, are generally viewed as standard "diet food." Thankfully, they're also popular party favorites and disappear quickly at almost any gathering. They add beauty, elegance, and color to any table or buffet and are the perfect complement to your favorite dip or pâté. Stuff a container or bag full of them to enjoy as a ready-to-eat snack when you are away from home.

2 carrots, sliced diagonally about ¼ inch (5 mm) thick

2 stalks celery, cut in half lengthwise and sliced into 3- to 4-inch (8- to 10-cm) pieces

1 cup (250 mL) whole sugar snap peas, trimmed

½ cucumber, sliced diagonally about ¼ inch (5 mm) thick

1 red bell pepper, cut lengthwise into eighths

1 green onion, cut into a flower (see sidebar)

1. Arrange the carrots, celery, sugar snap peas, cucumber, and bell pepper attractively on a platter.

2. Drain the green onion flower and use it to decorate the platter just before serving.

3. Serve immediately with Salsa Fresca (page 139), Sprouted Chickpea Hummus (page 141), or another dip, spread, or pâté of your choice.

How to Make a Green Onion Flower

To make a green onion flower, slice off and discard the roots from the end (the white tip) of the green onion with a sharp paring knife. Cut off most of the green portion of the shoots (reserve them for another use), leaving just a 2-inch (5-cm) length, measuring from the white tip. With the same knife, make a ½-inch-long (1-cm-long) slice into the white tip end of the onion, being very careful to penetrate only halfway (to the inside center). Rotate the onion, continuing to slice until you have 10–12 evenly spaced, paper-thin slices around the tip. Put the onion in ice water for 1 hour to allow the "petals" to open and form a flower.

kale coleslaw

The cabbage family includes Asian leaf vegetables such as bok choy and Napa cabbage, broccoli, Brussels sprouts, cauliflower, collards, kale, and kohlrabi. Today, cabbage is most widely consumed as coleslaw and is an all-American favorite. This easy-to-make, delicious, nutritious coleslaw combines both kale and cabbage. It is a popular standard at the Living Light Café and Cuisine To Go.

DRESSING

1 tablespoon (15 mL) freshly squeezed orange juice

1 tablespoon (15 mL) light miso

2 teaspoons (10 mL) flaxseed oil

1½ teaspoons (7 mL) agave syrup

1 teaspoon (5 mL) freshly squeezed lemon juice

1 teaspoon (5 mL) onion powder

1 teaspoon (5 mL) ground flaxseeds

1 small clove garlic, crushed

Pinch of powdered mustard

SALAD

2 cups (500 mL) kale leaves cut into thin ribbons

1¼ cups (310 mL) shredded cabbage

1 large ripe tomato, diced

½ cup (120 mL) mung bean or lentil sprouts

2 tablespoons (30 mL) red onion, finely julienned

½ red jalapeño chile, seeded and minced, or pinch of cayenne

Pinch of salt

1. For the dressing, combine all of the dressing ingredients in a large bowl and whisk until well blended.

2. Add the kale to the dressing and toss. Massage the kale well for a few minutes to soften. The kale should take on a "cooked" appearance and reduce dramatically in volume.

3. Add the cabbage, tomato, sprouts, onion, and chile and toss well. Season with salt to taste and toss again.

4. Kale Coleslaw is best served immediately, but it can also be stored in a covered container in the refrigerator for up 24 hours.

NUTRITION NOTE Kale is an extraordinary vegetable—among the most nutrient dense of all foods. Not surprisingly, one serving of this slaw provides over 100% of the RDA for vitamins C and K; over 40% of the RDA for vitamin A; over 20% of the RDA for chromium, folate, manganese, and vitamin B_6; and over 10% of the RDA for calcium, iron, magnesium, niacin, potassium, thiamin, vitamin E, and zinc.

kale and bok choy slaw with spicy sesame-ginger dressing

YIELD: 4 CUPS/1 L (3–4 SERVINGS)

The distinctively Asian flavors of this dish make it the perfect complement for Vegetable Sushimaki with Spicy Miso Paste (page 204), Vietnamese Salad Rolls (page 205), or any Asian-inspired meal.

SPICY SESAME-GINGER DRESSING

¼ cup (60 mL) raw tahini

1 tablespoon (15 mL) purified water

1 tablespoon (15 mL) light miso

1 tablespoon (15 mL) freshly squeezed lemon juice

1 tablespoon (15 mL) agave syrup

2 teaspoons (10 mL) grated fresh ginger

1 teaspoon (5 mL) onion powder

¼ teaspoon (1 mL) powdered mustard

¼ teaspoon (1 mL) salt

1 small clove garlic, crushed

Pinch of cayenne

SALAD

2 cups (500 mL) kale leaves, firmly packed, cut into thin ribbons

1¾ cups (430 mL) thinly sliced bok choy, packed

1 tomato, finely diced

1 apple, finely diced

½ cup (120 mL) mung bean or lentil sprouts

1½ tablespoons (22 mL) finely diced red onion

1. For the dressing, combine all of the dressing ingredients in a small bowl and whisk until well blended.

2. Place the kale in a large bowl and massage it well for a few minutes to soften. The kale should take on a "cooked" appearance and reduce dramatically in volume.

3. Add the remaining salad ingredients to the kale. Then add the dressing and toss well.

4. Kale and Bok Choy Slaw is best served within 3 hours, but it can also be stored in a covered container in the refrigerator for up 24 hours. The slaw will release some liquid when it is stored, but it will still taste good.

NUTRITION NOTE A serving of this lively salad provides 8 grams of protein, more than 20% of your day's supply of calcium, five B vitamins (folate, niacin, riboflavin, thiamin, and vitamin B_6), and fiber, plus all the vitamins C and K and beta-carotene you'll need for the day. It's a good source of iron and zinc too.

green garden salad bar

Many raw food enthusiasts enjoy a daily bountiful salad and never tire of it. This recipe makes a bright, colorful buffet meal all by itself. With this one salad and a variety of dressings, you can enjoy a different salad every day of the week. Be creative—try grated beets, broccoli, cauliflower, kale, spinach, watermelon radish, or any other veggies your heart desires.

¼ pound (114 g) baby greens

1½ ripe avocados, sliced lengthwise into quarters

½ head romaine lettuce, torn

¾ cup (180 mL) alfalfa sprouts

½ cup (120 mL) cherry tomatoes

½ cup (120 mL) mung bean or lentil sprouts

½ cucumber, sliced

½ red bell pepper, sliced

¼ cup (60 mL) sun-dried olives, rinsed well and pitted (optional)

¼ cup (60 mL) sunflower seeds

¼ cup (60 mL) pumpkin seeds

¼ cup (60 mL) shredded carrot

½ cup (120 mL) green onion, thinly sliced

Place each ingredient in a separate dish and arrange the dishes buffet style so everyone can create their own salad.

NUTRITION NOTE One serving of this salad provides 12 grams of protein, 11 grams of fiber, and over 20% of the RDA for nine vitamins (A, C, K, B_1, B_2, B_3, B_6, folate, and pantothenic acid) and seven minerals (copper, iron, magnesium, manganese, phosphorus, potassium, and zinc).

caesar salad with creamy horseradish dressing

YIELD: 6 SERVINGS

One of the most popular salads on any menu is the Caesar. Traditionally, its crisp romaine lettuce leaves are thickly coated in a redolent dressing and topped with crispy, crunchy croutons and sprinkled generously with fragrant Parmesan cheese. Unfortunately, Caesar salad almost always contains anchovies, making it unacceptable for vegetarians, in addition to the eggs in the dressing and cheese, which are unacceptable for vegans. Here's a fabulous Caesar with a horseradish dressing that contains all the components of the traditional salad except the animal products. This could very well be the best Caesar you have ever had!

CREAMY HORSERADISH DRESSING

1 cup (250 mL) peeled and chopped zucchini

¼ cup (60 mL) freshly squeezed lemon juice

3 tablespoons (45 mL) light miso

1 tablespoon (15 mL) grated fresh horseradish

2 teaspoons (10 mL) agave syrup

1½ teaspoons (7 mL) dulse flakes

½ teaspoon (2 mL) ground flaxseeds

1 clove garlic

Pinch of salt

Pinch of freshly ground white pepper

1 tablespoon (15 mL) flaxseed oil

SALAD

1 head romaine lettuce, torn or cut into pieces

1 cup (250 mL) Garlic-Herb Croutons (page 125; optional)

½ cup (120 mL) Pine Nut Parmesan (page 137; optional)

Freshly ground black pepper

1. For the dressing, combine the zucchini, lemon juice, miso, horseradish, agave syrup, dulse flakes, flaxseeds, garlic, salt, and white pepper in a blender and process until creamy.

2. With the blender running, slowly add the oil until the mixture is emulsified.

3. Place the lettuce in a large salad bowl, pour the dressing to taste over it, and toss. Sprinkle with the Garlic-Herb Croutons and Pine Nut Parmesan, if using. Add black pepper to taste, toss again, and serve immediately.

4. Stored in a sealed glass jar in the refrigerator, leftover Creamy Horseradish Dressing will keep for up to 4 days.

NUTRITION NOTE This Caesar salad may be the most nourishing version you could eat, with 13 grams of protein and over 40% of the RDA for three B vitamins (B_6, riboflavin, and thiamin) and vitamin C.

apples and walnuts on baby greens with poppy seed dressing

Pictured on p. 173

Pictured on p. 173

YIELD: 2-3 SERVINGS

This is a favorite holiday salad, reminiscent of Waldorf salad with the apples, celery, and nuts, but a refreshing change from the traditional version, which is heavy with mayonnaise. It is an outstanding source of omega-3 fatty acids. Poppy seeds and orange juice give it a special touch that pleases children as well as the sophisticated tastes of adults.

POPPY SEED DRESSING

2 tablespoons (30 mL) freshly squeezed orange juice

1 tablespoon (15 mL) flaxseed oil

1½ teaspoons (7 mL) Dijon mustard

½ teaspoon (2 mL) poppy seeds

½ teaspoon (2 mL) orange zest

Pinch of salt

SALAD

1½ red apples, diced

¼ cup (60 mL) walnuts, soaked and dehydrated (see page 64)

¼ cup (60 mL) thinly sliced celery

½ pound (225 g) baby greens

¼ cup (60 mL) pomegranate seeds (optional)

1. For the dressing, combine all of the dressing ingredients in a large bowl and whisk until well blended.

2. Add the apples, walnuts, celery, and pomegranate seeds, if using, and toss well.

3. Arrange the greens attractively on a platter, heap the apple mixture on top, and serve immediately.

variation: For extra flavor, replace the flaxseed oil with an equal amount of Omega Nutrition's Orange Flax Oil Blend.

vine-ripened heirloom tomatoes with fresh herbs

The hearty flavor and fresh appearance of this beautiful dish, combined with its ease of preparation, makes it a joy to serve. When they are in season, heirloom tomatoes are beyond compare. This dish makes a delightful appetizer or a fabulous complement to any meal. Serve it as is for a fat-free side dish or add Sweet Dijon Dressing (page 148).

1½ cups (370 mL) arugula, or ½ pound (220 g) fresh garden greens

3 large ripe heirloom tomatoes, very thinly sliced

Pinch of salt

1 tablespoon (15 mL) minced fresh herbs of your choice

1. Line a platter with the arugula and arrange the tomatoes over it.

2. Sprinkle with the salt and herbs. Serve immediately.

NUTRITION NOTE Tomatoes are a great source of chromium, which is known to enhance the action of insulin. One serving of this recipe provides 62% of the RDA for chromium.

"braised" spinach with mustard lemongrette

When prepared properly, braised greens have a fabulous flavor that is almost addictive. This recipe mimics the taste and texture of braised greens, and many people even prefer it!

MUSTARD LEMONGRETTE

1 tablespoon (15 mL) flaxseed oil

1 tablespoon (15 mL) light miso

2 teaspoons (10 mL) freshly squeezed lemon juice

2 teaspoons (10 mL) minced red onion

2 teaspoons (10 mL) agave syrup

1½ teaspoons (7 mL) Dijon mustard

¼ teaspoon (1 mL) salt

Pinch of freshly ground black pepper

SALAD

6 cups (1.5 L) baby spinach, packed

1½ tablespoons (22 mL) pine nuts

1. For the dressing, combine all of the dressing ingredients in a blender and process until smooth.

2. Place the spinach in a large bowl, add the dressing, and toss. Massage it well for a few minutes to soften. The spinach should take on a "cooked" appearance and reduce dramatically in volume.

3. To serve, mound each serving onto an individual plate and garnish with the pine nuts. Serve immediately.

NUTRITION NOTE A single serving of "Braised" Spinach with Mustard Lemongrette supplies over 30% of the RDA for folate, manganese, and vitamin A, and over 300% of the RDA for vitamin K!

sea vegetable and cucumber salad

YIELD: 1½ CUPS/370 ML (2–3 SERVINGS)

ea vegetables are a valuable asset to any diet due to their rich mineral content. Just soak them in water and watch them expand to many times their dried volume. This delightful salad combines tender sea vegetables with crispy cucumber and carrot and the pungent flavors of ginger, garlic, and chile—all of which add to the balance of this distinctive dish.

½ ounce (14 g) dried sea vegetables of your choice (such as arame, hijiki, sea palm, wakame), soaked in 1 cup (250 mL) purified water for 1 hour

1 carrot, shredded

½ cucumber, seeded and finely julienned

½ green onion, sliced

1 tablespoon (15 mL) raw sesame oil

1 tablespoon (15 mL) freshly squeezed lemon juice

1 tablespoon (15 mL) tamari

1½ teaspoons (7 mL) Ginger Juice (see sidebar)

1½ teaspoons (7 mL) sesame seeds

1 clove garlic, finely minced

½ teaspoon (2 mL) garlic powder

¼ teaspoon (1 mL) Hot Lava Sauce (page 171), or pinch of cayenne

¼ teaspoon (1 mL) toasted sesame oil

1. Drain the sea vegetables (reserve the water for plants or discard), rinse, and drain well again. Dry the sea vegetables between clean dish towels or paper towels. Cut into ½-inch (1-cm) pieces.

2. Transfer the sea vegetables to a medium bowl and add all of the remaining ingredients. Stir well until evenly combined.

3. Stored in an airtight container in the refrigerator, Sea Vegetable and Cucumber Salad will keep for up to 2 days.

ginger juice

To make small quantities of ginger juice, grate unpeeled fresh ginger using the fine side of a handheld grater. Put the grated ginger into a mesh strainer bag, a piece of cheesecloth, or a fine sieve and strain out the juice. Discard the pulp. To make a large quantity of ginger juice, a vegetable juicer may be used.

Stored in a sealed glass jar, Ginger Juice will keep for up to 1 week in the refrigerator. Alternatively, freeze Ginger Juice in ice cube trays. Once frozen, transfer the cubes to a sealed container. Frozen Ginger Juice will keep for up to 4 months.

dilled cucumbers

YIELD: 1½ CUPS/370 ML (3 SERVINGS)

Northern Europeans know that dill and cucumber were made for each other, and paired with a creamy cashew sauce, they never fail to please. This quick and easy recipe fits as perfectly into a picnic lunch as it does a gourmet dinner party.

3 cups (750 mL) peeled, seeded, and thinly sliced cucumbers

1½ teaspoons (7 mL) salt

6 tablespoons (90 mL) Cashew-Dill Sauce (page 158)

1. Place the cucumber slices in a large bowl with enough purified water to cover. Sprinkle the salt over the top of the cucumbers and set aside for 20–60 minutes. Rinse and drain well.

2. Gently toss the drained cucumbers with the Cashew-Dill Sauce and chill thoroughly before serving.

3. Stored in an airtight container in the refrigerator, Dilled Cucumbers will keep for up to 12 hours.

note: A mandoline (see page 97) is the perfect kitchen tool for creating thin, uniform cucumber slices.

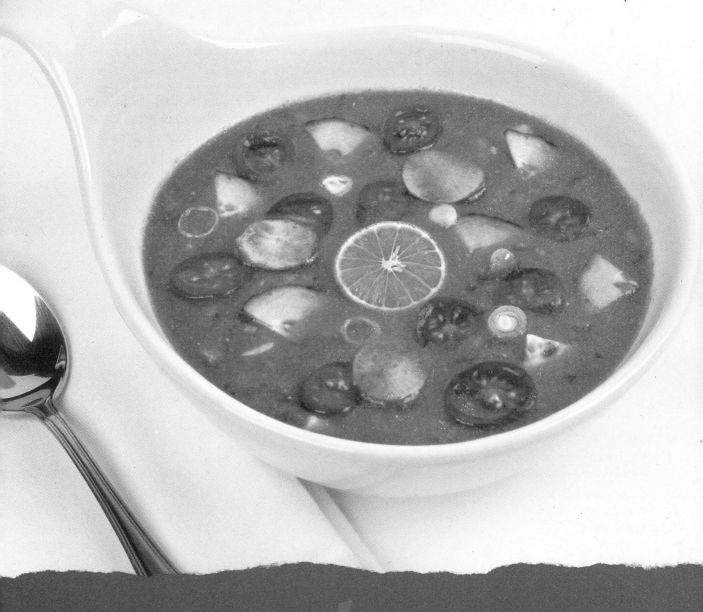

Gazpacho, p. 189

soups

SOUPS

creamy kale-apple soup

YIELD: 2½ CUPS/620 ML (1 HEARTY MEAL OR 2 SMALLER SERVINGS)

This soup is a mainstay for many raw food enthusiasts because of its simplicity, excellent flavor, and high nutritional content. You'll find this can be an almost daily favorite, with variations to suit your taste. The orange juice gives sweetness to the soup. For a less sweet soup, reduce or eliminate the orange juice and replace it with additional water or cucumber.

2 oranges, peeled and coarsely chopped

½ cup (120 mL) purified water

¼–⅓ cup (60–80 mL) sunflower seeds

4 cups (1 L) kale leaves, firmly packed

½ apple, chopped

½ green onion, coarsely chopped (optional)

1 tablespoon (15 mL) tamari

½ clove garlic, crushed

Pinch of cayenne

½ cup (120 mL) diced ripe tomatoes, or ½ apple, diced

2 tablespoons (30 mL) pumpkin or sunflower seeds (optional)

1. Combine the oranges, water, and sunflower seeds in a blender and process until completely smooth.
2. Add the kale, apple, optional green onion, tamari, garlic, and cayenne and process until thick and creamy.
3. Pour into soup bowls and garnish each serving with some of the tomatoes and a sprinkling of pumpkin seeds. Serve immediately.

variations: You can use a variety of vegetables in creamy green soups, such as bell pepper, celery, cucumber, fresh herbs, romaine lettuce, spinach, tomato, or zucchini. If you like, you can even add fresh fruits (in addition to or in place of the apple).

NUTRITION NOTE This soup is rich in vitamins and a multitude of minerals. The kale and seeds are abundant in calcium and protein; oranges further increase the calcium content.

fresh pea soup

Peas, in or out of the pod, are a protein-rich, low-fat addition to a raw diet. You may use either cold or hot water, depending on whether you want a cold or warm soup. Although frozen peas are not raw (they are blanched before they are frozen), they work well in this recipe if fresh peas are not available.

1 cup (250 mL) fresh or frozen peas

½ cup (120 mL) purified water

¼ small orange, coarsely chopped

2 teaspoons (10 mL) light miso

¼ teaspoon (1 mL) garlic powder

¼ teaspoon (1 mL) onion powder

Pinch of salt

Pinch of freshly ground white pepper

1 teaspoon (5 mL) chopped fresh dill weed or mint

2 teaspoons (10 mL) sunflower seeds (optional)

1. Combine the peas, water, orange, miso, garlic powder, onion powder, salt, and pepper in a blender and process until smooth and creamy.

2. Add the dill weed and pulse just until it is evenly incorporated.

3. Garnish with the optional sunflower seeds and serve immediately.

NUTRITION NOTE A serving of this delicious, creamy soup has only 1 gram of fat, yet it provides 10 grams of protein, plus it has more than one-quarter of your day's supply of beta-carotene, folate, niacin, thiamin, and vitamin K. It's also a good source of copper, iron, magnesium, and zinc.

garden blend soup

The vibrant green leaves of the kale plant provide an earthy flavor and offer more nutritional value per calorie than almost any other food. Vary the flavors of this soup to suit your taste; some people like it spicy and others like it sweet.

¾ cup (180 mL) purified water

¼ cup (60 mL) freshly squeezed orange juice, or ½ orange, coarsely chopped (see note)

3–4 cups (750 mL–1 L) chopped kale leaves, packed

½ apple, chopped, or ½ small cucumber, peeled and chopped

¼ cup (60 mL) fresh cilantro or basil leaves, or fresh dill weed, packed

1½ tablespoons (22 mL) light miso

1½ teaspoons (7 mL) freshly squeezed lemon juice

½ clove garlic

¼ red jalapeño chile, with seeds, or pinch of cayenne

½ green onion (optional)

¼ cup (60 mL) sunflower seeds, soaked for 1 hour, rinsed, and drained, or ½ ripe avocado, coarsely chopped

¼ cup (60 mL) mung bean sprouts, Spicy Sprouted Lentils (page 217), or Savory Seasoned Sunflower or Pumpkin Seeds (page 216)

1. Combine the water, orange juice, kale, apple, cilantro, miso, lemon juice, garlic, chile, and optional green onion (in this order) in a blender and process until smooth.

2. Add the sunflower seeds and process until smooth.

3. Garnish each serving with some of the sprouts and serve immediately.

variations

- You can use a variety of vegetables in garden soups, such as bell pepper, celery, cucumber, romaine lettuce, spinach, tomato, or zucchini.

- In cool months, use hot water for a warming soup.

note: The orange juice or orange gives sweetness to the soup. For a less sweet soup, reduce or eliminate the orange juice or orange and replace it with ¼ cup (60 mL) additional purified water or an additional ½ peeled cucumber, coarsely chopped.

NUTRITION NOTE A hearty, full-recipe serving of this soup will give you 17 grams of protein—one-third of your day's supply—plus an abundance of vitamins A, B (except for B_{12}), C, and E. It also supplies one-quarter of your calcium, iron, selenium, and zinc for the day, and all of your copper and manganese.

gazpacho

Pictured on p. 185

YIELD: 2 CUPS/500 ML (2 SERVINGS)

O n a hot day, there's nothing more refreshing than a cool bowl of Gazpacho soup. Traditionally served raw and cold or at room temperature, this soup makes great use of those perfectly ripe tomatoes from your garden. In the summer, when all of the vegetables are at their finest, this simple soup will be full of refreshing good flavor.

3 ripe tomatoes

¼ cup (60 mL) diced celery

¼ cup (60 mL) seeded and diced cucumber

3 tablespoons (45 mL) diced red bell pepper

2 teaspoons (10 mL) freshly squeezed lemon juice

¼ cup (60 mL) thinly sliced radishes

2 tablespoons (30 mL) minced fresh parsley, packed

1 tablespoon (15 mL) thinly sliced green onion

1½ teaspoons (7 mL) extra-virgin olive oil

½ teaspoon (2 mL) salt

Pinch of cayenne

Freshly ground black pepper

½ ripe avocado, diced

2 tablespoons (30 mL) Savory Seasoned Sunflower or Pumpkin Seeds (page 216), or ¼ cup (60 mL) mung bean sprouts or lentil sprouts (optional)

1. Seed the tomatoes and strain the seeds from the juice through a cloth mesh bag. Set the juice aside.

2. Finely dice the tomatoes.

3. Place the tomato juice, half of the celery, cucumber, and bell pepper, and all of the lemon juice in a blender and process until smooth.

4. Pour into a bowl and stir in the tomatoes, the remaining celery, cucumber, and bell pepper, and all of the radishes, parsley, green onion, oil, salt, cayenne, and black pepper. Chill in the refrigerator for at least 1 hour before serving.

5. Just before serving, stir in the avocado, pour into individual bowls, and top with the optional sunflower seeds.

6. Stored in a sealed glass jar in the refrigerator, Gazpacho will keep for up to 2 days.

NUTRITION NOTE Not surprisingly, Gazpacho is chock-full of nutrients and antioxidants. One serving of this soup supplies over 30% of the RDA for chromium, copper, magnesium, manganese, molybdenum, and vitamins B_6, C, and K, and over 20% of the RDA for pantothenic acid, potassium, and vitamins A and E.

minestrone italiano

This Italian favorite is so good it will have you saying *arrivederci* to traditional mine-strone. Cozy up with this mineral-rich soup for a comforting meal, served warm from the dehydrator or chilled and paired with Caesar Salad with Creamy Horseradish Dressing (page 178).

MARINATED VEGETABLES

¼ cup (60 mL) diced onion

½ cup (120 mL) freshly squeezed orange juice

1 tablespoon (15 mL) light miso

1½ teaspoons (7 mL) freshly squeezed lime juice

¼ cup (60 mL) diced zucchini

¼ cup (60 mL) diced red bell pepper

¼ cup (60 mL) thinly sliced celery

¼ cup (60 mL) diced carrot

¼ cup (60 mL) cut green beans (in 1-inch/2.5-cm pieces)

¼ cup (60 mL) small broccoli florets

¼ cup (60 mL) fresh or frozen corn kernels (see note)

¼ cup (60 mL) thinly sliced crimini mushrooms

2 tablespoons (30 mL) minced fresh parsley

½ teaspoon (2 mL) onion powder

½ clove garlic, crushed

SOUP STOCK

3 cups (750 mL) seeded and diced ripe tomatoes (reserve the seeds and juice in a small bowl)

¼ cup (60 mL) sun-dried tomatoes, soaked in 6 tablespoons (90 mL) purified water for 1 hour (do not drain)

2 teaspoons (10 mL) flaxseed oil

1½ teaspoons (7 mL) chopped fresh basil, or ½ teaspoon (2 mL) dried

¼ teaspoon (1 mL) Italian seasoning

Pinch of freshly ground black pepper

½ teaspoon (2 mL) salt

1. For the marinated vegetables, first remove the strong flavor from the onions by placing them in a strainer and rinsing them several times in purified water, squeezing them gently and rinsing them with fresh water each time.

2. Whisk the orange juice, miso and lime juice in a small bowl to blend. Transfer to an open glass jar or uncovered baking dish and add the onions and all of the remaining ingredients for the marinated vegetables. Dehydrate at 115 degrees F/45 degrees C for 1 hour to soften.

3. For the soup stock, put the reserved tomato seeds and juice and 1 cup (250 mL) of the diced tomatoes into a cloth mesh bag, and squeeze the bag into a medium bowl to strain the juice and separate it from the seeds. (Discard the seeds and pulp or add them to a blended soup or dressing.) Add the remaining 2 cups (500 mL) of diced tomatoes to the bowl of tomato juice.

4. Thinly slice the soaked sun-dried tomatoes and add them and their soaking water to the bowl with the tomatoes.

5. Add the oil, basil, Italian seasoning, and pepper and toss. Season with the salt to taste.

6. To serve, combine the warm marinated vegetables with the stock in a large bowl and stir. Serve warm from the dehydrator or chill until time to serve.

7. Stored in a sealed glass jar in the refrigerator, Minestrone Italiano will keep for up to 2 days.

note: Keep a supply of raw corn kernels on hand all year by buying plenty of summer corn and freezing it for the off-season. (Commercially frozen corn is blanched prior to packaging.) Simply remove the kernels from the cob and freeze small amounts in sealed containers. The corn will reduce in volume a bit, so allow a little extra for whatever recipe you have in mind; when defrosted, it will be the perfect amount. Frozen corn kernels will keep for up to 2–3 months.

NUTRITION NOTE With less than 150 calories per serving, Minestrone Italiano provides over 100% of the RDA for vitamin C and over 25% of the RDA for biotin, chromium, copper, molybdenum, niacin, potassium, and vitamin K.

spicy papaya soup

Savor the piquant combination of sweet, spicy, and tangy flavors in this exotic cream of papaya soup, served with a concassé (diced mixture) of avocado, cucumber, mango, and papaya, and drizzled with avocado crème fraiche. This recipe is one of Cherie's favorites and is the perfect starter to an elegant brunch.

SOUP

2½ cups (620 mL) coarsely chopped ripe papaya (about 1 medium-size papaya)

1 cucumber, peeled, seeded, and coarsely chopped

¾ cup (180 mL) purified water or coconut water

½ cup (120 mL) fresh cilantro, loosely packed

¼ cup (60 mL) freshly squeezed orange juice

1½ teaspoons (7 mL) freshly squeezed lime juice

4 teaspoons (20 mL) light miso

1½ teaspoons (7 mL) chopped onion

1 clove garlic, crushed

Pinch of cayenne, or ¼–½ teaspoon (1–2 mL) Hot Lava Sauce (page 171)

½ teaspoon (2 mL) ground cumin

¼ teaspoon (1 mL) salt

CONCASSÉ

¼ cup (60 mL) diced ripe avocado

¼ cup (60 mL) peeled, seeded, and diced cucumber

¼ cup (60 mL) diced ripe mango

¼ cup (60 mL) diced ripe papaya

GARNISH

½ ripe avocado

3 tablespoons (45 mL) purified water

¼ teaspoon (1 mL) salt

2 tablespoons (30 mL) minced red bell pepper

2 tablespoons (30 mL) minced fresh cilantro

1½ teaspoons (7 mL) Hot Lava Sauce (page 171)

1. For the soup, combine all of the soup ingredients in a blender and process until smooth.

2. For the concassé, combine all of the concassé ingredients in a medium bowl and toss gently.

3. To serve, place ¼ cup (60 mL) of the concassé in the center of individual soup bowls and carefully pour 1 cup (250 mL) of soup around the edge.

4. For the garnish, combine the avocado, water, and salt in a blender and process until smooth. Top each bowl with a dollop of the blended avocado, then sprinkle a little of the bell pepper, cilantro, and Hot Lava Sauce on top. Serve immediately.

NUTRITION NOTE Spicy Papaya Soup is a nutritional powerhouse with over 100% of the RDA for vitamins C and K and over 20% of the RDA for folate, pantothenic acid, potassium, and vitamin A.

tomato-mushroom bisque

What could be better on a cold winter evening than a bowl of warming soup? This robust bisque can be gently warmed in a dehydrator or on the stove top, as long as you keep a watchful eye on it. Alternatively, pour it into a glass jar and plunge it into hot water just before serving. As long as it is warmer than body temperature, it will be comforting to the spirit and warming to the body.

2 cups (500 mL) peeled and finely diced tomatoes

½ cup (120 mL) thinly sliced leek or green onions

½ cup (120 mL) finely diced celery

¼ cup (60 mL) diced zucchini

1 tablespoon (15 mL) chopped fresh dill weed

1 cup (250 mL) freshly squeezed orange juice

¼ cup (60 mL) pine nuts, soaked for 2 hours, rinsed, and drained

2 tablespoons (30 mL) Dried Shiitake Mushroom Powder (see page 164)

½ clove garlic, crushed

½ cup (120 mL) finely diced crimini mushrooms

½ teaspoon (2 mL) salt

¼ teaspoon (1 mL) truffle oil (optional)

Freshly ground black pepper

1. Combine half of the tomatoes, leek, celery, zucchini, and dill weed in a blender and add all of the orange juice, pine nuts, mushroom powder, and garlic. Process until smooth and creamy.

2. Pour into a large bowl and add the remaining tomatoes, leek, celery, zucchini, and dill weed, and the mushrooms, salt, optional truffle oil, and pepper to taste.

3. Serve at room temperature, chilled, or warmed in a dehydrator for 1 hour at 115 degrees F/45 degrees C.

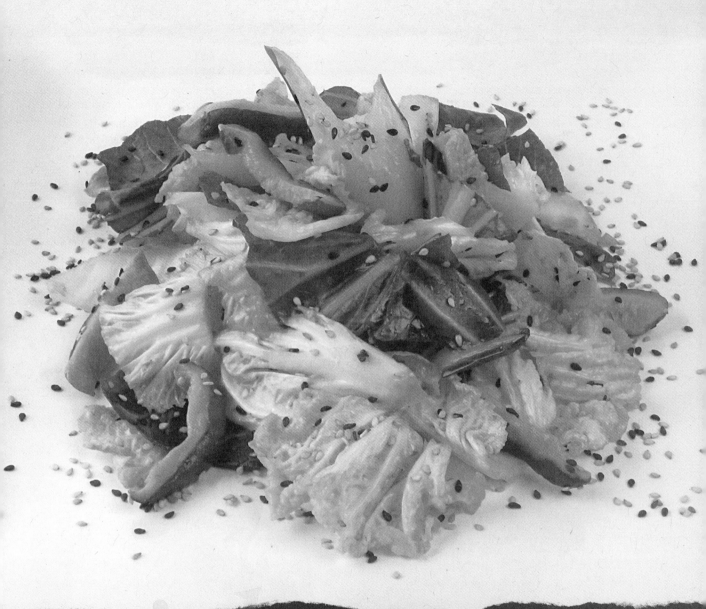

Baby Bok Choy with Shiitake
Mushrooms, p. 197

sides

SIDE DISHES

broccoli with bon bon sauce

When broccoli is at its peak of freshness, it's crisp and mild in flavor. When refrigerated for more than three to five days, it may look fine, but it becomes fibrous, woody, and strong tasting. One way of countering this aging process is to shock the broccoli with hot water. This softens it, brightens the color, and creates a milder flavor. The hot water just slightly warms the broccoli and then is poured off, so the broccoli is still crisp. It's divine with Bon Bon Sauce, although it is also delicious plain or in a salad once it has been shocked in this way.

5 cups (1.25 L) small broccoli florets

2 cups (500 mL) boiling purified water

1 cup (250 mL) Bon Bon Sauce (page 157)

1. Place the broccoli in a heatproof bowl and pour the boiling water over it. Keep the broccoli submerged for 1 minute, just long enough to remove the chill and turn the florets a brilliant green. Remove the broccoli from the water, immerse it in cold water, and drain well.

2. Pour the sauce over the broccoli and serve immediately.

3. Stored in a sealed container in the refrigerator, leftover Broccoli with Bon Bon Sauce will keep for up to 2 days.

note: Peel any leftover broccoli stems and use them for Crudités (page 174) or in salads and soups.

NUTRITION NOTE One serving of Broccoli with Bon Bon Sauce provides over 75% of the RDA for vitamin C, almost 50% of the RDA for thiamin, and over 25% of the RDA for zinc. It also provides a healthful dose of folate and trace minerals, as well as carotenoids and other antioxidants.

baby bok choy with shiitake mushrooms

Pictured on p. 195

YIELD: 6 CUPS/1.5 L (6 SERVINGS)

T his easy Asian side dish has become a staple at the Living Light Café and Cuisine To Go and is loved by our students for its simple yet balanced flavors. The few drops of toasted sesame oil add a distinct Asian flair and enhance its warmth and flavor.

3 quarts (3 L) baby bok choy

2 tablespoons (30 mL) raw sesame oil

2 tablespoons (30 mL) freshly squeezed lime juice

1 teaspoon (5 mL) salt

¼ teaspoon (1 mL) toasted sesame oil

1½ cups (370 mL) thinly sliced shiitake mushrooms

1. Separate the bok choy leaves and stack a few on top of each other. Slice the leaves lengthwise. (Smaller leaves should be cut in half widthwise; larger leaves should be cut into quarters.)

2. To make the marinade, whisk the raw sesame oil, lime juice, salt, and toasted sesame oil in a small bowl until well blended.

3. Combine the bok choy, mushrooms, and marinade in a large bowl and toss well. Cover and let marinate for 2–4 hours.

4. Drain and reserve the marinade and serve the salad immediately.

5. Stored in a sealed glass jar in the refrigerator, leftover marinade will keep for up to 4 days.

note: Use the leftover marinade in soups and dressings.

NUTRITION NOTE Bok choy is a mild, versatile vegetable and a good source of calcium and folic acid, important nutrients for pregnant women. Paired with the full-bodied, woodsy flavor of shiitake mushrooms, it's a unique and delightful combination. Shiitake mushrooms provide niacin, riboflavin, minerals such as copper, potassium, and selenium, and, when cultured outdoors in sunlight, vitamin D.

mexican-style seasoned cabbage

YIELD: 1½ CUPS/370 ML (3 SERVINGS)

This is one of the most popular dishes at the Living Light Café and Cuisine To Go and a favorite of our students. It was created to mimic Mexican seasoned rice, and it really does taste like the Spanish rice dishes served in Mexican restaurants. It's packed with nutrition, and since it tastes great, people come back for more.

1½ cups (370 mL) shredded cabbage (about ¼ head)

½–1 cup (120–250 mL) fresh or frozen peas (see notes)

1 green onion, thinly sliced

2 tablespoons (30 mL) Sun-Dried Tomato Powder (see page 129)

1 tablespoon (15 mL) extra-virgin olive oil

½ teaspoon (2 mL) salt

¼ teaspoon (1 mL) Mexican chili powder

¼ teaspoon (1 mL) ground cumin

¼ teaspoon (1 mL) onion powder

½ clove garlic, crushed

½ ripe tomato, diced

1. Place the cabbage in a food processor fitted with the S blade and pulse until it reaches the texture of rice.

2. Transfer to a large bowl and add the peas, green onion, Sun-Dried Tomato Powder, oil, salt, chili powder, cumin, onion powder, garlic, and tomato and toss gently.

3. If you would like to warm the mixture, transfer it to a large glass baking dish and place it in a dehydrator set at 125 degrees F/50 degrees C for 30 minutes to 2 hours, or in a warmed oven (preheated to warm and turned off) for 30 minutes prior to serving.

4. Serve immediately.

notes

- Frozen peas are not raw—they've been blanched for a few minutes. They still contain valuable nutrients as well as good flavor and color, but if you want a 100% raw recipe and have no fresh peas, they may be omitted.

- This dish is also tasty without being warmed. Try serving it wrapped in a large collard leaf or large leaf of romaine lettuce.

NUTRITION NOTE Thanks to the cabbage, this dish is high in vitamins C and K and the amino acid glutamine. Peas are a good source of protein and zinc.

vegetable antipasto

Serving fresh, lightly marinated vegetables as an antipasto (which means "before the meal") is a delicious way to tickle the taste buds of your guests. Be sure to purchase the vegetables at the height of their season (at their peak of ripeness and depth of flavor) and dress them fresh in salads or serve them as appetizers. As with all great art (food preparation included), simplicity can bring out the best, but it can also be challenging to do well. Once you've achieved a perfect balance of flavor, leave it alone. As they say, less is more. So when you have fresh, ripe vegetables, herbs, seasonings, and a little orange juice—*basta*. That's enough.

MARINADE

½ cup (120 mL) freshly squeezed orange juice (see note)

1 tablespoon (15 mL) freshly squeezed lemon juice

2 teaspoons (10 mL) flaxseed oil

1 teaspoon (5 mL) extra-virgin olive oil

1 teaspoon (5 mL) Italian seasoning

1 teaspoon (5 mL) powdered mustard

½ teaspoon (2 mL) salt

1 clove garlic, crushed

VEGETABLES

¼ pound (114 g) green beans, sliced lengthwise

1 zucchini, sliced crosswise

½ cup (120 mL) small cauliflower florets

½ cup (120 mL) small broccoli florets

4 medium-size mushrooms, sliced

½ red bell pepper, julienned

¼ leek, thinly sliced

1. For the marinade, combine all of the marinade ingredients in a small bowl and whisk to blend.

2. Combine the vegetables in a large bowl, add the marinade, and toss until evenly coated.

3. Transfer to glass jars and let marinate in the refrigerator for 8 hours. Alternatively, put the jars in a dehydrator and warm for 6 hours at 105 degrees F/40 degrees C (warming the vegetables in a dehydrator will help them to soften more quickly and better absorb the flavors of the marinade).

4. The vegetables may be served chilled, at room temperature, or warm (straight from the dehydrator). Remove them from the marinade with a slotted spoon and serve them with the marinade on the side.

5. Stored in an airtight container in the refrigerator, Vegetable Antipasto will keep for up to 2 days.

note: Orange juice adds sweetness to the marinade. For a less sweet taste, reduce the amount of orange juice.

wild rice pilaf

REQUIRES A DEHYDRATOR   **YIELD: 2 CUPS/500 ML (3 SERVINGS)**

It takes 24 hours to soften, or "bloom," wild rice, but when you want something filling and comforting, this savory, warm pilaf makes an excellent main dish or side dish at any meal, and it's a beautiful addition to your holiday feast. Wild rice is a marsh grass seed that is still harvested today by First Nations people and smoked according to their traditional methods. It's the smoking that allows it to "bloom," or fluff up without cooking. Even though wild rice is not technically raw, many raw food enthusiasts enjoy it and find it a very satisfying food. If you keep wild rice soaking in the refrigerator, you'll always have it handy for wild rice dishes any time the mood strikes.

½ cup (120 mL) wild rice

3 cups (750 mL) warm purified water

1 small stalk celery, diced

1 small carrot, shredded

½ cup (120 mL) lentil sprouts

1½ shiitake mushrooms, thinly sliced

1½ tablespoons (22 mL) chopped pecans

1½ tablespoons (22 mL) sunflower seeds

1½ tablespoons (22 mL) minced fresh parsley

½ green onion, sliced

1 teaspoon (5 mL) onion powder

1 teaspoon (5 mL) poultry seasoning

Pinch of garlic powder

1 tablespoon (15 mL) flaxseed oil

1½ teaspoons (7 mL) tamari

1 teaspoon (5 mL) dark miso

½ teaspoon (2 mL) freshly squeezed lemon juice

1. Place the rice in a glass jar and fill the jar to the top with the water. Cover the jar and place it in a dehydrator set at 105 degrees F/40 degrees C for 24 hours.

2. Rinse and drain the rice well and transfer it to a large bowl. Add the celery, carrot, sprouts, mushrooms, pecans, sunflower seeds, parsley, green onion, onion powder, poultry seasoning, and garlic powder and stir until well combined.

3. Combine the oil, tamari, miso, and lemon juice in a small bowl and stir until well combined. Pour over the rice mixture and stir until evenly distributed.

4. Stored in an airtight container in the refrigerator, Wild Rice Pilaf will keep for up to 4 days.

variations

ASIAN WILD RICE: Omit the lentil sprouts, pecans, sunflower seeds, and poultry seasoning. Add 1 tablespoon (15 mL) sesame seeds, 1 teaspoon (5 mL) toasted sesame oil, and 1 tablespoon (15 mL) Dried Shiitake Mushroom Powder (see page 164). For a little heat, season with cayenne to taste.

MEXICAN WILD RICE: Omit the lentil sprouts, pecans, sunflower seeds, and poultry seasoning. Add 1 cup (250 mL) diced ripe tomatoes, 2 tablespoons (30 mL) Sun-Dried Tomato Powder (see page 129), 1 teaspoon (5 mL) chili powder, ¼ teaspoon (1 mL) ground cumin, and cayenne to taste.

NUTRITION NOTE One serving of this pilaf boasts over 25% of the RDA for copper, manganese, niacin, vitamins A and K, and zinc.

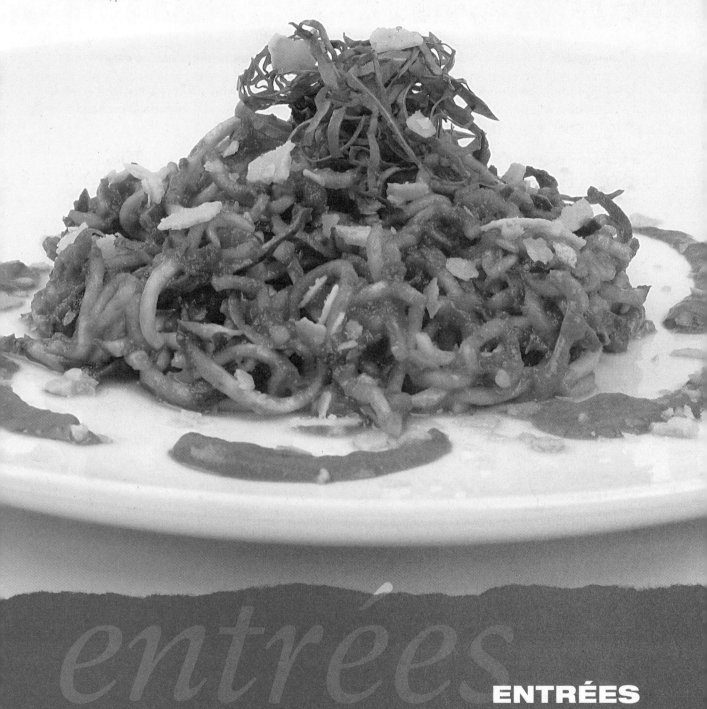

Zucchini Pasta with Pomodoro
Sauce, p. 210, and Pine Nut
Parmesan, p. 137

entrées

ENTRÉES

garden pizza

Pictured on p. 121

YIELD: 3 PIZZAS (3 SERVINGS)

rom the easy-to-make, crispy crust to the flavorful sauces, this pizza is a favorite staple of raw food enthusiasts. Make several pizza crusts in advance and have them on hand to enjoy whenever the mood for pizza strikes.

6 mushrooms, thinly sliced

½ teaspoon (2 mL) tamari

1½ teaspoons (7 mL) extra-virgin olive oil

3 Sprouted Seed Pizza Crusts (page 132) or Zucchini Pizza Crusts (page 131)

½ cup (120 mL) Pesto Sauce (page 162; optional)

½ cup (120 mL) Pizza Sauce (page 161; optional)

1½ ripe avocados, sliced lengthwise

7 Roma tomatoes, seeded and chopped

9 sun-dried olives, pitted and slivered (see note)

Pinch of salt (optional)

1. About 1 hour before assembling the pizza, toss the mushrooms in the tamari and oil and set aside.

2. To assemble the pizzas, drain the mushrooms and have all the remaining ingredients prepared and set aside.

3. Spread a layer of the optional Pesto Sauce and/or Pizza Sauce evenly on top of each crust. Add a layer of the avocado, tomatoes, mushrooms, and olives. If desired, sprinkle lightly with a little salt to taste. Serve immediately or warm in a dehydrator set at 115 degrees F/45 degrees C for up to 2 hours.

note: Sun-dried olives are very salty and will taste best if some of the salt is removed before they are used. Simply rinse them well, then cover them with twice the amount of water as olives. Add several cloves of crushed garlic and some minced fresh or dried Italian herbs. Allow the olives to soak in the refrigerator for 24 hours, then drain them well. Sun-dried olives will keep in a sealed glass jar in the refrigerator for up to 1 month.

mexican burritos

This Mexican standard is greatly appreciated by all fans of raw cuisine. It can be prepared simply, in very little time, by using romaine lettuce leaves to wrap up the filling. Or, for a more traditional burrito, take the time to make Fresh Corn Tortillas and enjoy a burrito that will impress even your Mexican friends. *Muy delicioso!*

FILLING

1 ripe avocado, mashed

1 small zucchini, diced

1 ripe tomato, seeded and diced

¼ cucumber, diced

¼ cup (60 mL) fresh or frozen corn kernels (see note, page 191)

¼ cup (60 mL) lentil sprouts

1 green onion, sliced

1 red Anaheim chile, seeded and diced, or ½ cup (120 mL) diced red bell pepper

1¼ cups (310 mL) finely shredded cabbage

2 tablespoons (30 mL) minced fresh cilantro

¼ teaspoon (1 mL) cayenne or Hot Lava Sauce (page 171)

¼ teaspoon (1 mL) salt

WRAPS

6 large romaine lettuce leaves, or 6 Fresh Corn Tortillas (page 126)

1. Combine all of the filling ingredients in a large bowl and stir until evenly mixed.

2. Spoon each serving into a single large lettuce leaf or tortilla, roll it up, and serve immediately.

3. Stored in an airtight container in the refrigerator, leftover filling will keep for up to 12 hours.

NUTRITION NOTE With only 290 calories per serving (when made with Fresh Corn Tortillas) and 22% of calories from fat, these burritos make a tasty, light meal. As a bonus, they're packed with antioxidants, minerals, and vitamins, and provide over 100% of the RDA for chromium, riboflavin, thiamin, and vitamins B_6 and C, and over 60% of the RDA for niacin, selenium, and vitamin K.

vegetable sushimaki with spicy miso paste

Nori, also called laver, is one of the most popular sea vegetables in the world and is very mild in flavor. Nori is dried in thin sheets, which are ideal for making sushi rolls, also known as maki or sushimaki. Maki can be filled with any combination of vegetables or fruits, so don't stop with this recipe—use your imagination! Vegetable Sushimaki with Spicy Miso Paste makes a great lunch paired with Sea Vegetable and Cucumber Salad (page 182), or serve it as an elegant appetizer for a Japanese meal.

SPICY MISO PASTE

2 tablespoons (30 mL) dark miso

1 tablespoon (15 mL) raw sesame oil (optional)

¾ teaspoon (4 mL) Hot Lava Sauce (page 171), or pinch of cayenne

SUSHIMAKI

6 sheets nori

9 cups (2.25 L) alfalfa sprouts

1½ ripe avocados, thinly sliced lengthwise

1 red bell pepper, julienned

½ cucumber, seeded and julienned

1 carrot, shredded

Optional Condiments

6 tablespoons (90 mL) tamari

1 tablespoon (15 mL) wasabi powder, mixed with purified water to form a thick paste

2 tablespoons (30 mL) sesame seeds

1. For the miso paste, combine the miso, optional sesame oil, and Hot Lava Sauce in a small bowl and stir well.

2. To make the sushimaki, lay one sheet of nori, shiny side down, on a bamboo sushi mat. Using the back of a teaspoon, lightly spread approximately 1 teaspoon (5 mL) of the miso paste over the nori sheet.

3. At the end of the nori sheet closest to you, layer some alfalfa sprouts, avocado, bell pepper, cucumber, and carrot. To roll the sushi, grip the edge of the nori sheet and the sushi mat with your thumbs and forefingers, and press the filling back with your other fingers. Using the mat to help you, roll the front end of the nori over the filling. Give it a squeeze with your mat, and then lift the forward edge of the mat and continue rolling the nori, using the mat to help compress the filling slightly. Seal the end of the nori roll with a little purified water.

4. Cut the roll into 8 pieces using a very sharp knife or a serrated knife.

5. Repeat these steps with the remaining 5 nori sheets.

6. Serve immediately with the optional tamari and/or wasabi paste, and garnish with the sesame seeds, if desired.

NUTRITION NOTE Vegetable Sushimaki with Spicy Miso Sauce is a wonderful source of antioxidants, including vitamins C and E, and a variety of carotenoids.

vietnamese salad rolls

These Vietnamese-inspired fresh spring rolls are even better than the originals! The rice papers, which are the traditional wrappers, can be purchased in any Asian market or replaced with cabbage leaves or paper-thin sheets of cucumber. The fresh vegetable filling is crowned with a piquant sesame-ginger sauce that is out of this world.

SAUCE

1 cup (250 mL) Bon Bon Sauce (page 157)

¼ teaspoon (1 mL) Thai red curry paste

SALAD ROLLS

6 rice paper wrappers or cabbage leaves (see note)

1 head green leaf lettuce

1 green onion, sliced

1 bunch cilantro, large stems removed

2 cups (500 mL) mung bean sprouts

1½ carrots, shredded

6–12 sprig fresh mint or Thai basil leaves

1. For the sauce, combine the Bon Bon Sauce and curry paste in a medium-size bowl and mix well.

2. For the salad rolls, moisten 2 of the rice paper wrappers and overlap them midway to form a straighter outer edge. Place 2 of the lettuce leaves horizontally, stem sides facing each other and the leafy ends sticking out, on the bottom half of the wrappers. Stack the remaining ingredients on top of the rice paper wrappers and lettuce leaves, beginning with some of the sauce. Roll up the salad roll (rolling both rice paper sheets in unison) and cut the roll in half crosswise. Repeat until all 3 rolls are complete.

3. Serve with the remaining sauce for dipping.

4. Stored in separate airtight containers in the refrigerator, Vietnamese Salad Rolls and sauce will keep for up to 1 day.

note: Use 8-inch (20-cm) round Vietnamese dried rice paper wrappers (*banh trang*). If you prefer a totally raw salad roll, since rice paper wrappers are not raw, replace them with 6 whole cabbage leaves.

NUTRITION NOTE The nutrient profile for these rolls is outstanding, with 16 grams of protein and 9 grams of fiber per serving, plus over 100% of the RDA for vitamins A, C, and K, and over 45% of the RDA for folate, iron, manganese, thiamin, and zinc (if eaten with cabbage leaf wrappers).

vegetable teriyaki stirred, not fried

Pictured on p. 147   **YIELD: 1 QUART (1 L) VEGETABLES PLUS 4 PINEAPPLE SKEWERS (6 SERVINGS)**

Teriyaki sauce is a combination of sweet, pungent, salty, and lively flavors, which make this dish irresistible. The aroma and flavor of this enticing sauce, combined with an abundance of fresh seasonal vegetables like bok choy, broccoli, peppers, and shiitake mushrooms, make it one of the most popular standards at the Living Light Café and Cuisine To Go. When the vegetables are marinated, they soften and take on the texture and appearance of cooked vegetables. This dish is good served with Wild Rice Pilaf (page 200) and Baby Bok Choy with Shiitake Mushrooms (page 197).

TERIYAKI MARINADE AND PINEAPPLE

¼ cup (60 mL) tamari

2 tablespoons (30 mL) evaporated cane juice

1½ tablespoons (22 mL) raw sesame oil

1½ tablespoons (22 mL) freshly squeezed lemon juice

1 tablespoon (15 mL) flaxseed oil or extra-virgin olive oil

1 tablespoon (15 mL) onion powder

3 cloves garlic, crushed

1 teaspoon (5 mL) grated fresh ginger

¼ teaspoon (1 mL) toasted sesame oil

¼ teaspoon (1 mL) freshly ground black pepper

¼ large pineapple, peeled, cored, and cubed

1. For the marinade, combine the tamari, evaporated cane juice, raw sesame oil, lemon juice, flaxseed oil, onion powder, garlic, ginger, toasted sesame oil, and pepper in a blender and process briefly, just until combined. (Do not overblend, as this will incorporate too much air.)

2. Arrange the pineapple in a shallow baking dish, pour the marinade over it, and toss. Let sit at room temperature while you prepare the vegetables.

3. Remove the pineapple from the marinade and place 4–6 pieces on 4 (6-inch/15-cm) skewers, leaving one end of each skewer free to use as a handle.

VEGETABLES

¾ cup (180 mL) snow peas, cut in half lengthwise

¾ cup (180 mL) thinly sliced shiitake mushrooms

¾ cup (180 mL) thinly sliced baby bok choy

¾ cup (180 mL) mung bean sprouts

½ cup (120 mL) finely chopped broccoli with stems

½ cup (120 mL) thinly sliced celery (sliced crosswise)

½ red bell pepper, finely julienned

½ carrot, finely julienned

¼ red onion, finely julienned

4. Combine the vegetables in a large bowl, add the marinade, and toss. Transfer to an unsealed glass jar and put it in a dehydrator set at 125 degrees F/50 degrees C for 30 minutes to 2 hours, or in a warmed oven (preheated to warm and turned off) for 30 minutes prior to serving. Alternatively, the vegetables can marinate in the refrigerator for 8–12 hours. Pour off the marinade before serving and reserve it for other uses, if desired (see note).

5. If you wish, place the pineapple skewers on a nonstick dehydrator sheet in the same warm dehydrator for 1–2 hours. Serve the pineapple skewers warm or at room temperature on top of the warm vegetables.

notes

- Use leftover marinade for sauces and salad dressings. Stored in a sealed glass jar in the refrigerator, the marinade will keep for up to 1 week.

- Leftover vegetables and pineapple can be dehydrated for 24 hours at 105 degrees F/40 degrees C and served as crunchy snacks.

zoom burgers

REQUIRES A DEHYDRATOR *Pictured on p. 165*   YIELD: 3-4 SMALL BURGERS

Unlike meat burgers, the flavor of Zoom (short for zucchini-mushroom) Burgers is outstanding on its own, even without all the trimmings. They can be served between Sprouted Grain Buns (page 122), regular burger buns, or wrapped in several leaves of romaine lettuce (our favorite) with lots of fresh tomatoes, thinly sliced onions, Real Tomato Ketchup (page 168), Cashew Mayonnaise (page 166), and Hot Mustard (page 167).

¾ cup (180 mL) walnuts, soaked and dehydrated (see page 64)

1 cup (250 mL) shredded zucchini

1 tablespoon (15 mL) dark miso

1 tablespoon (15 mL) purified water

¾ cup (180 mL) minced mushrooms

⅓ cup (80 mL) minced celery

¼ cup (60 mL) minced red onion

2 tablespoons (30 mL) ground flaxseeds

1½ tablespoons (22 mL) minced fresh parsley

1 tablespoon (15 mL) nutritional yeast flakes

1½ teaspoons (7 mL) minced fresh sage

½ teaspoon (2 mL) salt

1 clove garlic, crushed

¼ teaspoon (1 mL) freshly ground white pepper

1. Place ½ cup (120 mL) of the walnuts in a food processor fitted with the S blade and grind them into a powder. Add the zucchini and pulse to mix. (Do not overprocess; the mixture should have a little texture.) Transfer to a large bowl.

2. Mince the remaining walnuts by hand or coarsely grind them by pulsing them in the food processor.

3. Place the miso and water in a small bowl and stir them together with a fork to form a loose paste. Add the paste and all of the remaining ingredients to the zucchini mixture and stir well.

4. Form 3-4 small burger patties, each about ½ inch (1 cm) thick, using approximately ½ cup (120 mL) of the mixture per patty. (If smaller burgers are desired, use less of the mixture).

5. Place the burgers on a dehydrator tray lined with a nonstick sheet and dehydrate them at 105 degrees F/40 degrees C for 4 hours. Turn the burgers over onto a mesh dehydrator tray (without a nonstick sheet) and continue dehydrating for 2–8 hours longer, or until the outside is crusty and the inside is moist and chewy.

6. Stored in an airtight container in the refrigerator, Zoom Burgers will keep for up to 3 days.

variation

ZOOM CROQUETTES: For a more elegant dinner entrée, form the mixture into oval croquettes instead of burgers using ½ cup (120 mL) for each one. Top the dehydrated croquettes with Onion-Shiitake Gravy (page 164).

NUTRITION NOTE The walnut base in these burgers supplies a full day's supply of omega-3 fatty acids, and the nutritional yeast provides a bountiful boost of B vitamins.

zucchini pasta with basil pesto

YIELD: 3 CUPS/750 ML (3 SERVINGS)

Spiralized zucchini looks and satisfies like pasta. Its flavor is neutral, like traditional pasta, yet it's so much faster to prepare. Paired with fresh sweet basil, pungent garlic, and the richness of walnuts, this pasta with pesto sauce is to live for!

ZUCCHINI PASTA

4 zucchini

BASIL PESTO

½ cup (120 mL) chopped zucchini

1 cup (250 mL) fresh basil leaves, firmly packed

1 tablespoon (15 mL) flaxseed oil

1½ teaspoons (7 mL) light miso

1½ teaspoons (7 mL) nutritional yeast flakes

1 clove garlic

Pinch of salt

¼ cup (60 mL) walnuts

GARNISH

1½ tablespoons (22 mL) Pine Nut Parmesan (page 137)

Freshly ground black pepper

1. For the pasta, transform the zucchini into noodles using a spiral slicer (see page 87).

2. For the pesto, place the chopped zucchini in a food processor fitted with the S blade and process until smooth. Add the basil, oil, miso, nutritional yeast flakes, garlic, and salt and pulse a few times to coarsely chop the basil. Add the walnuts and process until the desired consistency is achieved. Do not overprocess or the oil from the walnuts will separate and the mixture will become too oily. The texture should be creamy, with tiny specks of walnuts throughout.

3. Add the pesto to the Zucchini Pasta and toss lightly. Serve topped with the Pine Nut Parmesan and pepper to taste.

4. Stored in a sealed glass jar in the refrigerator, leftover Basil Pesto will keep for up to 4 days.

zucchini pasta with pomodoro sauce

Pictured on p. 201

YIELD: 4 CUPS/1 L (3 SERVINGS)

Pasta fresca! Pomodoro sauce is a fresh tomato sauce that is chunkier than the typically thick, rich marinara that simmered all day on Grandma's stove. In fact, "pomodoro" is simply the Italian word for tomato. This lively pasta sauce is fresh and flavorful and can be made in minutes. We suggest putting it over spiralized zucchini, but any kind of squash or root vegetables will do. Turnips, rainbow beets, celery root, or rutabaga all make great angel hair pasta for pomodoro.

ZUCCHINI PASTA

6 zucchini

POMODORO SAUCE

3 Roma tomatoes, seeded and chopped

¼ cup (60 mL) Sun-Dried Tomato Powder (see page 129)

1½ tablespoons (22 mL) finely minced onion

1 tablespoon (15 mL) extra-virgin olive oil

1 tablespoon (15 mL) minced fresh basil leaves

1½ teaspoons (7 mL) minced fresh oregano

1 clove garlic, crushed

¼ teaspoon (1 mL) salt

Pinch of freshly ground black pepper

Pinch of cayenne

GARNISH

3 tablespoons (45 mL) Pine Nut Parmesan (page 136)

Freshly ground black pepper

1. Transform the zucchini into noodles using a spiral slicer (see page 87).

2. To make the sauce, place the tomatoes in a colander to allow any liquid to drain. (Drink the wonderful juice or add it to another recipe.) When the tomatoes are thoroughly drained, transfer them to a food processor fitted with the S blade and pulse briefly to create a chunky sauce. (Do not overprocess; the tomatoes should have some texture.)

3. Add the Sun-Dried Tomato Powder, onion, olive oil, basil, oregano, garlic, salt, pepper, and cayenne and pulse briefly to mix.

4. Allow the sauce to sit for 10 minutes to thicken before you serve it.

5. Serve the Zucchini Pasta on individual plates with a generous scoop of Pomodoro Sauce on top. Garnish with the Pine Nut Parmesan and black pepper to taste.

6. Stored in a sealed glass jar in the refrigerator, leftover Pomodoro Sauce will keep for up to 3 days.

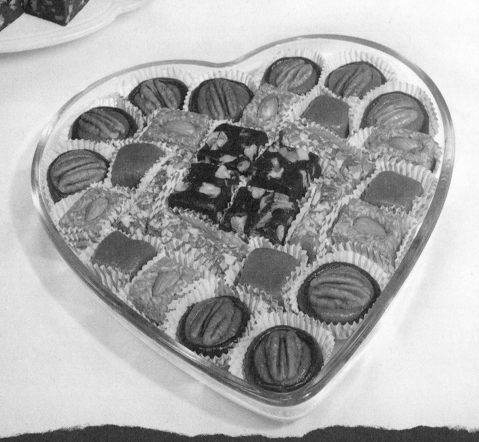

Turtle Truffles and variations, p. 213

sweets

SNACKS AND SWEETS

figgie nut'ins

YIELD: ABOUT 30 COOKIES (15 SERVINGS)

F iggie Nut'ins are a perfect sweet snack for all ages. They can be varied to create any number of deliciously flavored cookies and piecrusts, and they can be formed into different shapes. Eat them when they are soft and chewy, or dehydrate them until they are crunchy (which makes them store well for traveling, since no refrigeration is needed). No-bake nut cookies are great for holiday entertaining and make excellent gifts that can be safely mailed. Figgie Nut'ins and other cookies and brownies made from nuts and dried fruit freeze well. Children like making them and sharing them with their friends. It might just make your kids more interested in eating nutritious foods!

2 cups (500 mL) almonds, soaked for 8 hours, rinsed, and drained

3 cups (750 mL) dried figs, stems removed, chopped, soaked in warm purified water for 5 minutes, and well drained

1½ cups (370 mL) walnuts, soaked for 8 hours, rinsed, and drained

½ teaspoon (2 mL) orange zest

1. Place the almonds in a food processor fitted with the S blade and grind into a meal. Add the figs, walnuts, and orange zest and process until well combined. The mixture should stick together when pressed firmly in your palm.

2. Form the mixture into small balls using 2 tablespoons (30 mL) per ball, and flatten them with your hand to make cookies that are about ½ inch (1 cm) thick and 3 inches (8 cm) in diameter.

3. Eat the cookies soft as is, or dehydrate them at 105 degrees F/40 degrees C on a dehydrator tray lined with a nonstick sheet for 4–24 hours, depending on how soft and moist you want them.

4. Stored in an airtight container, Figgie Nut'ins will keep for up to 1 month in the refrigerator or up to 4 months in the freezer.

variations

Instead of forming the mixture into cookies, enjoy it straight from the bowl.

SWEET NUT'INS: Replace the figs with an equal amount of any chopped dried fruit you prefer. Especially delicious are apricots, blueberries, cherries, cranberries, or dates.

CHOCOLATE (OR CAROB) FIGGIE NUT'INS: Add 2 tablespoons (30 mL) of unsweetened raw cocoa powder or carob powder during processing.

NUTRITION NOTE These sweet treats will not only give you an energy boost; they also deliver 7 grams of protein and 1.2 grams of omega-3 fatty acids per serving (2 cookies), plus the minerals calcium, iron, magnesium, and zinc.

turtle truffles

Pictured on p. 211

YIELD: ABOUT 30 TRUFFLES (12 SERVINGS)

These hand-rolled truffles seem like they should be breaking some raw food law, they are so deliciously rich. They're for special occasions and celebrations; even though they are far better for you than traditional sugar candies, they're not something to eat daily. If you enjoy them occasionally and in moderation, though, you don't have to feel guilty eating these divine truffles.

CARAMEL

1 cup (250 mL) pitted soft dates, packed

1 cup (250 mL) pine nuts

½ teaspoon (2 mL) vanilla extract

FUDGE

1 cup (250 mL) pitted soft dates, packed

½ cup (120 mL) raisins or dried cherries

6 tablespoons (90 mL) almond butter

⅔ cup (160 mL) unsweetened cocoa or carob powder

Pinch of ground cinnamon

GARNISH

½ cup (120 mL) unblemished pecan halves

1. For the caramel, loosely separate the dates and place them in a food processor fitted with the S blade. Add the pine nuts and vanilla extract and process until smooth. Transfer the mixture to a glass container and place in the freezer while making the fudge.

2. For the fudge, loosely separate the dates and place them in the same food processor (no need to clean the work bowl). Add the raisins and almond butter and process until smooth. Add the cocoa powder and cinnamon and process again until evenly incorporated.

3. Roll the caramel into balls, using 1 teaspoon (5 mL) of the mixture for each one. Do the same for the fudge, also using 1 teaspoon (5 mL) of the mixture for each ball.

4. Using your thumb, make a depression in the center of a ball of fudge large enough to fit a ball of caramel inside.

5. Holding the two balls together (the ball of caramel inside the ball of fudge), carefully pull the fudge up around the caramel to create a coating, and press a pecan half on top. Repeat this process until all the truffles are formed. Refrigerate them for at least 1 hour before serving.

6. Serve each truffle in a paper candy cup.

7. Stored in an airtight container in the refrigerator or freezer, Turtle Truffles will keep for up to 1 month.

variation

ASSORTED CANDIES: Use the Caramel and Fudge separately or with the addition of chopped nuts or shredded coconut to form a variety of candies.

lemon and herb seaflower snacks

REQUIRES A DEHYDRATOR

YIELD: 24 ROLLS (6 SERVINGS)

These crunchy, slightly salty, health-promoting snacks are fun to make and great to take on road trips.

1 cup (250 mL) sunflower seeds, soaked for 4 hours, rinsed, and drained

3 tablespoons (45 mL) freshly squeezed lemon juice

½ teaspoon (2 mL) Italian seasoning

½ teaspoon (2 mL) dried basil

1 clove garlic, crushed

¼ teaspoon (1 mL) salt

¼ teaspoon (1 mL) freshly ground black pepper

Pinch of lemon zest

Pinch of freshly ground white pepper

6 nori sheets, cut into quarters

1. Process the soaked sunflower seeds in a food processor fitted with the S blade or a Champion or Green Star Juicer fitted with the homogenizing plate and grind them into a smooth paste.

2. Transfer to a medium-size bowl and add the lemon juice, Italian seasoning, basil, garlic, salt, black pepper, lemon zest, and white pepper. Mix well.

3. Using 1½ teaspoons (7 mL) of the mixture, form a long cylindrical roll along the length of the quarter sheet of nori near the side closest to you.

4. Roll the nori jelly-roll style and seal the edge with a few drops of purified water.

5. Repeat this process with all of the remaining nori sheets.

6. Place the rolls on a dehydrator tray and dehydrate at 105 degrees F/40 degrees C for about 48 hours, or until they are completely dry.

7. Stored in a tightly sealed glass jar in a cool place or in the refrigerator, Lemon and Herb Seaflower Snacks will keep for up to 2 months.

NUTRITION NOTE Besides being a delicious snack, sunflower seeds are high in magnesium, selenium, and vitamin E.

pure power bars

These tasty, power-packed bars make a great midmorning snack or travel companion. Don't be put off by the fact that they contain sea vegetables. If anything will make you fall in love with sea vegetables, this could be it! If they are to be used as a travel snack, they can be dehydrated, or eat them as is—soft and chewy.

3 cups (750 mL) chopped figs

3 cups (750 mL) warm purified water

1 cup (250 mL) almonds, soaked for 8 hours, rinsed, and drained

1 cup (250 mL) Brazil nuts, soaked for 8 hours, rinsed, and drained

1 cup (250 mL) walnuts, soaked for 3 hours, rinsed, and drained

3 cups (750 mL) sesame seeds, soaked for 3 hours, rinsed, and drained

1 cup (250 mL) pumpkin seeds, soaked for 3 hours, rinsed, and drained

¼ cup (60 mL) dulse flakes

2 tablespoons (30 mL) ground cinnamon

1½ cups (370 mL) ground flaxseeds

1 cup (250 mL) dried blueberries

1½ cups (370 mL) agave syrup

1. Soak the figs in the warm water for 20 minutes. Transfer the figs and their soaking water to a blender and process into a paste.

2. Rinse and drain all the seeds and nuts and allow them to air-dry for 2 hours. Place the almonds, Brazil nuts, and walnuts in a food processor fitted with the S blade and grind them into a fine meal.

3. Add the sesame seeds, pumpkin seeds, dulse, and cinnamon and pulse briefly. Do not overprocess; the mixture should have bits of seeds visible.

4. Transfer the mixture to a large bowl. Add the flaxseeds and blueberries and stir well. Stir in the agave syrup, mixing until it is evenly incorporated.

5. Dehydrating the bars is optional. To dehydrate them, spread 6 cups (1.5 L) of the mixture evenly on each of 2 dehydrator trays lined with nonstick sheets, and carefully score each one into 32 bars. (Score into 4 long strips in one direction and 8 strips in the opposite direction, forming 32 rectangular bars.) Using a second dehydrator tray without a nonstick liner, flip the tray over and remove the nonstick sheet to allow complete airflow. Dehydrate at 105 degrees F/40 degrees C for 18–24 hours.

7. Stored in a sealed container in the refrigerator, dehydrated Pure Power Bars will keep for up to 2 months; if the bars are not dehydrated, they will keep for up to 2 weeks.

variation: For a chunkier texture, chop the walnuts and add them with the flaxseeds and blueberries.

NUTRITION NOTE These delicious bars are filled with calcium-rich seeds and have many nutrients that tend to be hard to obtain, like iodine, selenium, and zinc. The dulse in this recipe provides your day's supply of iodine in a serving (2 bars). However, if you have another source of iodine, such as iodized salt or a supplement, you can omit it and still have an excellent, nutrient-rich bar.

savory seasoned sunflower or pumpkin seeds

This snappy snack is a great additions to soups and salads.

6 cups (1.5 L) sunflower or pumpkin seeds, soaked 4–6 hours, rinsed, and drained

⅓ cup (80 mL) tamari

1 tablespoon (15 mL) onion powder

½ teaspoon (2 mL) garlic powder

¼ teaspoon (1 mL) cayenne

1. Combine all of the ingredients in a medium-size bowl and stir to mix.

2. Spread the seeds on mesh dehydrator trays (use a scant 2 cups/ 500 mL per tray). Dehydrate at 105 degrees F/40 degrees C for 18–24 hours, or until crisp.

3. Stored in an airtight container in the refrigerator, Savory Seasoned Sunflower or Pumpkin Seeds will keep for up to 6 months.

NUTRITION NOTE Sunflower seeds are high in iron, phosphorous, potassium, protein, and zinc and are a great source of vitamin E. Pumpkin seeds are an excellent source of trace minerals, especially iron, magnesium, manganese, and zinc. They also provide high-quality protein and healthful fats.

spicy sprouted lentils

REQUIRES A DEHYDRATOR   YIELD: 4 CUPS/1 L (16 SERVINGS)

Seasoned, lightly dehydrated sprouted lentils are low in fat and high in protein. They make a convenient, chewy snack and add interest to salads at home or when you go out to eat.

6 cups (1.5 L) sprouted lentils

3 tablespoons (45 mL) tamari

1 tablespoon (15 mL) curry powder

2 teaspoons (10 mL) onion powder

¼ teaspoon (1 mL) garlic powder

Pinch of cayenne

1. Combine all of the ingredients in a medium-size bowl and stir to mix.

2. Spread the lentil sprouts on mesh dehydrator trays (use a scant 2 cups/500 mL per tray). Dehydrate at 105 degrees F/40 degrees C for 3–4 hours, or until they are lightly dried but still chewy. Take care that they don't become overly dehydrated and crunchy or they'll be difficult to chew.

3. Stored in an airtight container in the refrigerator, Spicy Sprouted Lentils will keep for up to 2 weeks.

NUTRITION NOTE Lentils are an excellent source of folate and magnesium, making them heart healthy as well as good for your waistline. They also provide low-cost, high-quality protein. Sprinkle these sprouts liberally on soups and salads or just use them in place of nuts when snacking for a low-fat treat.

falafel chickpea nuts

Also known as garbanzo beans, chickpeas are buttery, nutty-tasting legumes that provide a delicious source of protein that's lower in fat than nuts or seeds yet satisfying and crunchy. Chickpeas are used in Latin American, Italian, Indian, and Middle Eastern cooking. Falafel Chickpea Nuts make a convenient, chewy snack and add interest to salads at home or when you go out to eat. Try adding different seasonings to make a variety of flavors.

6 cups (1.5 L) sprouted chickpeas

¼ cup (60 mL) light miso

2 teaspoons (10 mL) onion powder

2 teaspoons (10 mL) ground coriander

2 teaspoons (10 mL) ground cumin

1 teaspoon (5 mL) garlic powder

¼ teaspoon (1 mL) cayenne

1. Combine all of the ingredients in a medium-size bowl and stir to mix.

2. Spread the chickpea sprouts on mesh dehydrator trays (use a scant 2 cups/500 mL per tray). Dehydrate at 105 degrees F/40 degrees C for 3–4 hours, or until they are lightly dried but still soft and chewy.

3. Stored in an airtight container in the refrigerator, Falafel Chickpea Nuts will keep for up to 2 weeks.

almost oatmeal cookies

REQUIRES A DEHYDRATOR   **YIELD: ABOUT 24 SMALL COOKIES (10–12 SERVINGS)**

These taste so much like traditional oatmeal cookies, people will argue that they must be! These no-bake cookies are easy enough for kids to make and they love them. This recipe can be varied in many ways and even used as a pressed cookie crust for fresh fruit pies.

1½ cups (370 mL) chopped pitted dates, packed

1½ cups (370 mL) almonds, soaked for 12–24 hours, rinsed, and drained

1 cup (250 mL) walnuts, soaked for 8–12 hours, rinsed, and drained

2 teaspoons (10 mL) ground cinnamon

½ teaspoon (2 mL) vanilla extract

½ cup (120 mL) raisins

½ cup (120 mL) walnuts, soaked, dehydrated, and chopped

See Soaked and Dehydrated Nuts, page 64

1. Loosely separate the dates and place them in a food processor fitted with the S blade. Add the almonds, the 1 cup (250 mL) soaked walnuts, and all of the cinnamon and vanilla extract. Process until the mixture begins to stick together.

2. Transfer to a large bowl, add the raisins and the ½ cup (120 mL) dehydrated walnuts, and stir well.

3. Form the dough into round cookies about ¼ inch (5 mm) thick and 2 inches (5 cm) in diameter.

4. Place the cookies on a dehydrator tray lined with a nonstick sheet and dehydrate at 105 degrees F/40 degrees C for 12–36 hours, until the desired texture is obtained. Turn the cookies over and remove the nonstick sheet after about 6 hours.

5. Stored in an airtight container, Almost Oatmeal Cookies will keep for up to 1 month in the refrigerator or up to 4 months in the freezer.

variations

MAPLE-WALNUT COOKIES: Omit the raisins and replace the vanilla extract with maple flavoring.

CHOCOLATE CHIP COOKIES: Omit the raisins and add ½ cup (120 mL) of nondairy chocolate or carob chips.

bananas! I scream

This ice cream tastes rich and delicious, but it is 100% fruit, nondairy, and guilt free! It's perfect for children and adults alike. Serve it with Chocolate Velvet (page 221) or Fruit Coulis (page 222) and you'll have the perfect summer treat.

5 ripe bananas, peeled and frozen (see note)

1. Run the frozen bananas through a Champion or Green Star Juicer fitted with the homogenizing plate. Alternatively, break the bananas into chunks and process them in a food processor fitted with the S blade until smooth.

2. Serve immediately. Stored in a sealed container in the freezer, Bananas! I Scream will keep for several hours before it freezes solid, making it impossible to serve. Once frozen solid, it will need to thaw slightly before serving.

note: Store frozen bananas in a sealed container in the freezer for up to 2 months.

chocolate velvet

YIELD: 1½ CUPS/370 ML (6-8 SERVINGS)

Chocolate is a source of antioxidants, but it can be very addictive, so use it sparingly. This sauce is velvety smooth and creamy and will feed the soul of even the fussiest chocolate lover. The secret ingredient, avocado, makes it thick and rich, but it cannot be detected in the flavor. Use Chocolate Velvet as a topping for Bananas! I Scream (page 220) or other desserts, or serve it on its own as a pudding.

1 ripe avocado

6 tablespoons (90 mL) unsweetened raw cocoa powder or carob powder

¼ cup (60 mL) agave syrup

2 tablespoons (30 mL) evaporated cane juice

½ cup (120 mL) plus 2 tablespoons (30 mL) purified water

½ teaspoon (2 mL) vanilla extract

Pinch of ground cinnamon

1. Combine the avocado, cocoa powder, agave syrup, evaporated cane juice, 2 tablespoons (30 mL) of the water, and all of the vanilla extract and cinnamon in a food processor fitted with the S blade and process until smooth.

2. Add the remaining ½ cup (120 mL) of water and process again until well blended. The more water you add, the thinner the sauce will be. (If you prefer to use a blender rather than a food processor, be careful not to process the mixture too long. If too much air is beaten into the sauce it will become too fluffy.)

3. Stored in a sealed glass jar in the refrigerator, Chocolate Velvet will keep for up to 1 week.

variations

CHOCOLATE FROSTING OR FILLING: Use only 2 tablespoons (30 mL) of the water and omit the remaining ½ cup (120 mL).

CHOCOLATE MOUSSE: Use a blender instead of a food processor and use only ¼ cup (60 mL) of the water to create a fluffy consistency similar to a classic mousse.

FROZEN FUDGE BARS: Freeze the mixture in Popsicle trays.

fruit coulis

Coulis is a French term referring to a thick sauce made of puréed fruit or vegetables. Even though coulis is most often made from berries, any fresh or frozen juicy fruit can be used to create a sauce that's lovely served with raw vegan ice cream, fruit pie, fruit salad, or anything chocolate. Try berry, cherry, peach, pineapple, or even tomato coulis!

2 cups (500 mL) fresh or frozen fruit

1 cup (250 mL) pitted dates or other dried fruit, packed

1. Place the fruit in a blender with a small amount of purified water and process until smooth.

2. Loosely separate the dates and add them to the blender. Process until smooth. (Sweeter fruit will require fewer dates.) If your dates are very dry, process them for a minute, then turn the blender off and allow the dates to remain in the puréed fruit for a few minutes to soften. Continue processing until smooth.

3. Stored in a sealed glass jar in the refrigerator, Fruit Coulis will keep for up to 4 days.

NUTRITION NOTE All berries are good sources of phytochemicals and vitamin C. In fact, just 6–8 strawberries provide all the vitamin C you need for an entire day!

apple pie with carob-pecan crust

The taste and smell of cinnamon and apples has long been a favorite of North Americans and Europeans alike. This no-bake apple pie will satisfy the need for one of our favorite comfort foods. The recipe was entered into a "cooked" pie contest and beat out all its competition. No worries about sacrificing flavor with this people pleaser!

CRUST

1½ cups (370 mL) pecans, soaked and dehydrated (see page 64)

1 cup (250 mL) chopped dried figs (see note)

¼ cup (60 mL) unsweetened raw carob powder

FILLING

6 apples, shredded

¾ cup (180 mL) dried apples, packed and ground (see note)

2 tablespoons (30 mL) evaporated cane juice

1 teaspoon (5 mL) ground cinnamon

Pinch of ground nutmeg

TOPPING

1½ cups (370 mL) Sweet Cashew Cream (page 107)

1. To make the crust, place the pecans, figs, and carob powder in a food processor fitted with the S blade and process until the mixture holds together easily. Press into an 8-inch (20-cm) pie pan.

2. For the filling, combine the fresh apples, dried apples, evaporated cane juice, cinnamon, and nutmeg in a large bowl and stir well or mix with your hands.

3. Press the filling firmly into the crust. Serve with Sweet Cashew Cream.

4. Stored in a sealed container in the refrigerator, Apple Pie with Carob-Pecan Crust will keep for up to 3 days.

notes

- If the figs are very dry, soak them in purified water to cover for 10 minutes, then drain well.

- To grind dried apples or pineapple, first snip the dried fruit with kitchen shears, then grind the pieces in a food processor fitted with the S blade.

banana-fig pudding

This pudding is surprisingly delicious and takes only a few minutes to make. It's fat free and will satisfy that desire for a sweet treat in the afternoon or evening. Keep dried figs soaking in purified water in the refrigerator to snack on or use in desserts any time the mood strikes.

2 large ripe bananas

8 dried figs, soaked for 2 hours

Pinch of ground cinnamon

1. Combine all of the ingredients in a blender and process until smooth and creamy.

2. Eat immediately or chill in the refrigerator before serving (the pudding will get thicker and firmer as it chills). Stored in a sealed container in the refrigerator, Banana-Fig Pudding will keep for up to 3 days.

NUTRITION NOTE Each serving of Banana-Fig Pudding provides 13 grams of fiber and about 100 mg of calcium.

apricot-apple compote

YIELD: 6 SERVINGS

This simple, delicious compote will evoke memories of Grandma's home cooking. Enjoy it plain as a pudding or top it with Fruit Coulis (page 222).

24 dried apricot halves, soaked for 4 hours and drained

4 apples, peeled and chopped

½ cup (120 mL) pitted dates

2 teaspoons (10 mL) peeled and grated fresh ginger

½ teaspoon (2 mL) ground cinnamon

8 fresh ripe apricots, diced

1. Combine the dried apricots, apples, dates, ginger, and cinnamon in a blender and process until smooth.
2. Fold in the fresh apricots.
3. Chill the compote in the refrigerator for 1 hour or longer before serving.
4. To serve, divide the compote equally among glass serving cups or shallow wine glasses.
5. Stored in a sealed container in the refrigerator, Apricot-Apple Compote will keep for up to 3 days.

carob-banana pudding

Don't be surprised if this delicious, easy-to-make pudding becomes a favorite for breakfast as well as dessert. Eat it alone or layer it with fruit for a spectacular parfait.

6 large ripe bananas

6 large pitted prunes

⅓ cup (80 mL) unsweetened raw carob powder

2 tablespoons (30 mL) molasses or evaporated cane juice

2 teaspoons (10 mL) vanilla extract

½ teaspoon (2 mL) ground cinnamon

Pinch of salt

1. Combine all of the ingredients in a blender and process until smooth and creamy.

2. Chill the pudding in the refrigerator for 1 hour or longer before serving.

3. Stored in a sealed container in the refrigerator, Carob-Banana Pudding will keep for up to 3 days.

APPENDIX 1 Dietary Reference Intakes (DRI) for Vitamins*

Life Stage/Age	Vit A[a] mcg	Vit C mg	Vit D[b] mcg	Vit E mg	Vit K mcg	Thiamin mg	Ribo-flavin mg	Niacin[c] mg	Vit B6 mg	Folate[d] mcg	Vit B12[e] mcg	Pantothenic Acid mg	Biotin mcg	Choline mg
INFANTS														
0–6 months	400	40	5	4	2.0	0.2	0.3	2	0.1	65	0.4	1.7	5	125
7–12 months	500	50	5	5	2.5	0.3	0.4	4	0.3	80	0.5	1.8	6	150
CHILDREN														
1–3 years	**300**	**15**	5	**6**	30	**0.5**	**0.5**	**6**	**0.5**	**150**	**0.9**	2	8	200
4–8 years	**400**	**25**	5	**7**	55	**0.6**	**0.6**	**8**	**0.6**	**200**	**1.2**	3	12	250
MALES														
9–13 years	**600**	**45**	5	**11**	60	**0.9**	**0.9**	**12**	**1**	**300**	**1.8**	4	20	375
14–18 years	**900**	**75**	5	**15**	75	**1.2**	**1.3**	**16**	**1.3**	**400**	**2.4**	5	25	550
19–30 years	**900**	**90**	5	**15**	120	**1.2**	**1.3**	**16**	**1.3**	**400**	**2.4**	5	30	550
31–50 years	**900**	**90**	5	**15**	120	**1.2**	**1.3**	**16**	**1.3**	**400**	**2.4**	5	30	550
51–70 years	**900**	**90**	10	**15**	120	**1.2**	**1.3**	**16**	**1.7**	**400**	**2.4**	5	30	550
>70 years	**900**	**90**	15	**15**	120	**1.2**	**1.3**	**16**	**1.7**	**400**	**2.4**	5	30	550
FEMALES														
9–13 years	**600**	**45**	5	**11**	60	**0.9**	**0.9**	**12**	**1**	**300**	**1.8**	4	20	375
14–18 years	**700**	**65**	5	**15**	75	**1.0**	**1.0**	**14**	**1.2**	**400**	**2.4**	5	25	400
19–30 years	**700**	**75**	5	**15**	90	**1.1**	**1.1**	**14**	**1.3**	**400**	**2.4**	5	30	425
31–50 years	**700**	**75**	5	**15**	90	**1.1**	**1.1**	**14**	**1.3**	**400**	**2.4**	5	30	425
51–70 years	**700**	**75**	10	**15**	90	**1.1**	**1.1**	**14**	**1.5**	**400**	**2.4**	5	30	425
>70 years	**700**	**75**	15	**15**	90	**1.1**	**1.1**	**14**	**1.5**	**400**	**2.4**	5	30	425
PREGNANCY														
18 years	**750**	**80**	5	**15**	75	**1.4**	**1.4**	**18**	**1.9**	**600**	**2.6**	6	30	450
19–30 years	**770**	**85**	5	**15**	90	**1.4**	**1.4**	**18**	**1.9**	**600**	**2.6**	6	30	450
31–50 years	**770**	**85**	5	**15**	90	**1.4**	**1.4**	**18**	**1.9**	**600**	**2.6**	6	30	450
LACTATION														
18 years	**1,200**	**115**	5	**19**	75	**1.4**	**1.6**	**17**	**2**	**500**	**2.8**	7	35	550
19–30 years	**1,300**	**120**	5	**19**	90	**1.4**	**1.6**	**17**	**2**	**500**	**2.8**	7	35	550
31–50 years	**1,300**	**120**	5	**19**	90	**1.4**	**1.6**	**17**	**2**	**500**	**2.8**	7	35	550

*Recommended Dietary Allowances (RDAs) are in **bold type** and Adequate Intakes (AIs) are in regular type. Both RDA and AI can be used as goals for individual intake.

Source: Food and Nutrition Board, The Institute of Nutrition, National Academies of Sciences. DRI reports can be accessed free at www.nap.edu (Search for "Dietary Reference Intakes" and several books will be shown—all can be opened online and read free of charge).

[a] Vitamin A: as retinal activity equivalents (RAEs); 1 RAE = 1 μg retinol; 12 μg beta-carotene, 24 μg other pro-vitamin A carotenoids in foods

[b] Vitamin D: 1 μg cholecalciferol = 40 IU vitamin D

[c] Niacin: as niacin equivalents (NE); 1 mg of niacin = 60 mg tryptophan; 0–6 months must receive preformed niacin, not NE

[d] Folate: as dietary folate equivalents (DFE); 1 DFE = 1 μg food folate = 0.6 μg of folic acid from fortified food or supplement consumed with food, or 0.5 μg of supplement consumed on an empty stomach

[e] Vitamin B12: 10–30% of people 50 years of age and older have poor absorption of vitamin B12; thus they are advised to meet the RDA using B12-fortified foods or supplements

APPENDIX 2 Dietary Reference Intakes (DRI) for Minerals

Life Stage/Age	Calcium mg	Chromium mcg	Copper mcg	Fluoride mg	Iodine mcg	Iron mg	Magnesium mg	Manganese mg	Molybdenum mcg	Phosphorus mg	Selenium mcg	Zinc mg
INFANTS												
0–6 months	210	0.2	200	0.01	110	0.27	30	0.003	2	100	15	2
7–12 months	270	5.5	220	0.5	130	11	75	0.6	3	275	20	3
CHILDREN												
1–3 years	500	11	340	0.7	90	7	80	1.2	17	460	20	3
4–8 years	800	15	440	1	90	10	130	1.5	22	500	30	5
MALES												
9–13 years	1,300	25	700	2	120	8	240	19.0	34	1,250	40	8
14–18 years	1,300	35	890	3	150	11	410	2.2	43	1,250	55	11
19–30 years	1,000	35	900	4	150	8	400	2.3	45	700	55	11
31–50 years	1,000	35	900	4	150	8	420	2.3	45	700	55	11
51–70 years	1,200	30	900	4	150	8	420	2.3	45	700	55	11
>70 years	1,200	30	900	4	150	8	420	2.3	45	700	55	11
FEMALES												
9–13 years	1,300	21	700	2	120	8	240	1.6	34	1,250	40	8
14–18 years	1,300	24	890	3	150	15	360	1.6	43	1,250	55	9
19–30 years	1,000	25	900	3	150	18	310	1.8	45	700	55	8
31–50 years	1,000	25	900	3	150	18	320	1.8	45	700	55	8
51–70 years	1,200	20	900	3	150	8	320	1.8	45	700	55	8
>70 years	1,200	20	900	3	150	8	320	1.8	45	700	55	8
PREGNANCY												
≤18 years	1,300	29	1,000	3	220	27	400	2.0	50	1,250	60	13
19–30 years	1,000	30	1,000	3	220	27	350	2.0	50	700	60	11
31–50 years	1,000	30	1,000	3	220	27	360	2.0	50	700	60	11
LACTATION												
≤18 years	1,300	44	1,300	3	290	10	360	2.6	50	1,250	70	14
19–30 years	1,000	45	1,300	3	290	9	310	2.6	50	700	70	12
31–50 years	1,000	45	1,300	3	290	9	320	2.6	50	700	70	12

* Recommended Dietary Allowance (RDA) is in **bold type** and Adequate Intake (AI) is in regular type. Both RDA and AI can be used as goals for individual intake.

Source: Food and Nutrition Board, The Institute of Nutrition, National Academies of Sciences. DRI reports can be accessed free at www.nap.edu (Search for "Dietary Reference Intakes" and several books will be shown—all can be opened online and read free of charge).

RawRevolutionDiet.com

RawRevolutionDiet.com is the companion website for this book. Here you will find additional information to support your goals and your personal revolution, including additional recipes, case histories, testimonials, articles, nutritional information, sprouting information, sprouting charts, press releases, author appearance schedules, and resource guides. Be sure to visit this dynamic website regularly for the latest Raw Food Revolution Diet news.

Raw Culinary Training, Supplies, and Prepared Food

www.RawFoodChef.com

Info@RawFoodChef.com
301-B North Main Street, Fort Bragg, CA 95437 USA
Phone: 707-964-2420

Living Light Culinary Arts Institute: Provides expert training in raw vegan cuisine for individuals, chefs, and teachers. Curriculum covers everything from sprouting to gourmet cuisine and professional certification.

Living Light Marketplace: Retail and online store for culinary supplies, including: juicers, dehydrators, spiral slicers, high-powered blenders, knives, culinary videos, specialty foods, organic body care, and books.

Living Light Café and Cuisine To Go: Award-winning organic vegan café and deli offers smoothies, juices, wraps, salads, soups, entrées, desserts, and various ethnic dishes. Open seven days a week.

Living Light Inn: Eco-friendly lodging on the Mendocino coast. Raw vegan kitchen, full-house water filtration, composting, nontoxic cleaning supplies, and more. Walking distance from Living Light Center.

Nutrition Consultation with Registered Dietitians

Brenda Davis, RD

www.brendadavisrd.com
brendadavis@telus.net
1094 Lambeth Court, Kelowna, BC V1V 1N2 Canada

Vesanto Melina, MS, RD

www.nutrispeak.com
vesanto@nutrispeak.com
Phone: 604-882-6782
20543 96th Ave, #34, Langley BC, V1M 3W3 Canada

Brenda Davis and Vesanto Melina provide nutritional consultation to those on raw food, vegan, and vegetarian diets, and those in transition. They have expertise in weight management, prevention and treatment of chronic diseases such as heart disease, and fine-tuning plant-based diets during pregnancy, infancy, childhood, and throughout life. Brenda Davis has special expertise in diabetes, and Vesanto Melina in food sensitivities. Consultations are available by a combination of phone and e-mail, or in their offices. Brenda Davis and Vesanto Melina are dynamic, internationally acclaimed presenters, and are available to speak at your event.

other books by the authors

Angel Foods: *Healthy Recipes for Heavenly Bodies*. Cherie Soria. Book Publishing Company, 2003.

Becoming Vegan. Brenda Davis and Vesanto Melina. Book Publishing Company, 2000.

Becoming Vegetarian. Vesanto Melina and Brenda Davis. Wiley Canada, 2003 (in Canada).

Comiendo Pura Vida. Cherie Soria and Rodrigo Crespo. Heartstar Productions, 2002.

Defeating Diabetes. Brenda Davis and Tom Barnard, MD. Book Publishing Company, 2003.

Food Allergy Survival Guide. Vesanto Melina, Jo Stepaniak, and Dina Aronson. Healthy Living Publications, 2004.

The New Becoming Vegetarian. Vesanto Melina and Brenda Davis. Book Publishing Company, 2003.

Raising Vegetarian Children. Jo Stepaniak and Vesanto Melina. McGraw-Hill, 2003.

iron, 58–59, 228
I Scream, Bananas!, 220
Italian Herb Dressing, 150
Italiano, Minestrone, 190–91

J
jalapeño chiles, in *Spicy Sweet-and-Sour Sauce,* 160
Jam, Berry-Date, 169
journal. *See* diet and lifestyle record
juice
   ginger, 183
   Green Giant, 119
   kale, 119
   V-5, 120
juicers, 85–86
   types of, 86
juicing, 61–62

K
kale, 175
   -Apple Soup, Creamy, 186
   in *Blue-Green Smoothie for One,* 103
   and Bok Choy Slaw with Spicy Sesame-Ginger Dressing, 176
   Coleslaw, 175
   in *Garden Blend Soup,* 188
   in *Green Giant Juice,* 119
   juicing, 119
   sprouting, 90
   in *V-5 Juice,* 120
kamut/kamut berries
   about 73
   in *Multi-Grain Cereal,* 122
   in *Sprouted Grain Bread,* 122
   in *Sprouted Multi-Grain Bread,* 123
kelp powder, in *Not Salmon/Tuna Salad,* 146
Ketchup, Real Tomato, 168
kitchen
   cleaning out, 69–70
   replacing old favorites with healthy alternatives, 70
   saving time in the, 76–78
kitchen tools, 78–89
knives and other cutting tools, 86–87
Kraut, Cabbage, 170

L
Lava Sauce, Hot, 171
laver (nori), in *Vegetable Sushimaki with Spicy Miso Paste,* 204
legumes, 23–24, 73
   calories and protein in, 41
   sprouting, 90
lemon
   -Ginger Sauce, Mangoes in, 110

-grette, "Braised" Spinach with Mustard, 181
-grette, Pineapple, 152
and Herb Seaflower Snacks, 214
lentil(s)
   blood sugar and, 142
   cholesterol and, 142
   iron in, 142
   Pâté with Garlic and Herbs, Sprouted, 142
   Spicy Sprouted, 217
   sprouting, 90
leptin, 4
lettuce, in *Green Giant Juice,* 119
lifestyle, 31, 33
Lime Cocktail, Gingery Apple-, 116
Liquid Gold Dressing, 151
Living Light Culinary Arts Institute, xiii, xvi, 229
locally grown food. *See* farmers' markets
lutein, 49
lycopene, 49

M
Macadamia Nut Cheese, 137
macadamia nuts, as variation, in *Cashew Yogurt,* 108
magnesium, 59, 228
mandoline, 87
manganese, 59, 228
mango(es), 110
   in *Lemon-Ginger Sauce,* 110
   -Pineapple Smoothie, 105
   Salad, Banana-, 109
   in *Spicy Sweet-and-Sour Sauce,* 160
Maple-Walnut Cookies, 219
marinade(s)
   Italian Herb Dressing, 150
   Pineapple Teriyaki Sauce, 159
   Sweet Dijon Dressing, 148
   for *Vegetable Antipasto,* 199
   for *Vegetable Teriyaki Stirred, Not Fried,* 206–7
Marinara Sauce, 163
Mayonnaise, Cashew, 166
meals, 28
Mexican recipes
   Burritos, 203
   Corn and Avocado Salsa, 140
   Fresh Corn Tortillas, 126
   Seasoned Cabbage, 198
   Wild Rice, 200
millet, in *Sprouted Multi-Grain Bread,* 123
mindful eating, 28

minerals, 54–59
   probiotics to increase absorption of, 108
mineral supplements, 29
   as safety measure, 60
Minestrone Italiano, 190–91
miso, 73–74
Miso Nut Cheese, 137
Miso Paste, Vegetable Sushimaki with Spicy, 204
molybdenum, 59, 228
Mousse, Chocolate, 221
Multi-Grain Cereal, 112
multivitamins, 29
   as safety measure, 60
mushroom(s)
   Baby Bok Choy with Shiitake, 197
   Bisque, Tomato-, 193
   Powder, Dried Shiitake, 164
   in *Zoom Burgers,* 208
   in *Zoom Croquettes,* 208
Mustard, Hot, 167
Mustard Lemongrette, "Braised" Spinach with, 181

N
niacin, 52, 227
nori (laver), in *Vegetable Sushimaki with Spicy Miso Paste,* 204
Not Salmon Salad, 146
Not Tuna Salad, 146
nut(s). *See also* specific types of
   calories and protein in, 40–41
   Cheese, Basic, 136
   Cheese, Miso, 137
   dehydrated, 64
   inclusion in a raw diet, 24–25
   'ins, Chocolate (or Carob) Figgie, 212
   'ins, Figgie, 212
   'ins, Sweet, 212
   and nut butters, 74
   soaking, 63–64, 111, 138
   sprouting, 90
   as variation, in *Cashew Yogurt,* 108

O
oat(s)
   -meal, Cinnamon, 113
   -meal Cookies, Almost, 219
   in *Multi-Grain Cereal,* 112
obesity, defined, 7
obesity battle, 1–2
   emotional factors, 4–5
   environmental factors, 3
   physical factors, 2–4

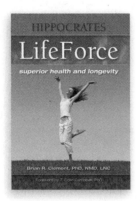
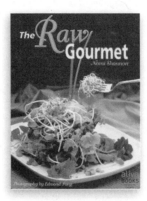
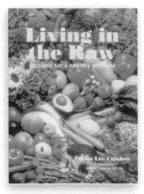
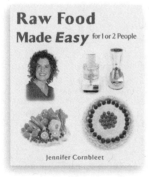
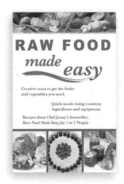
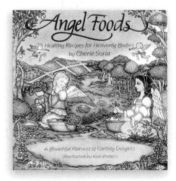